Student Workbook for

The Administrative Dental Assistant

Third Edition

Linda J. Gaylor, RDA, BPA, MEd
Coordinator, Curriculum and Instruction
San Bernardino County Superintendent of Schools
Regional Occupational Program, Career Training, and Support Services
San Bernardino, California

ELSEVIER
SAUNDERS

ELSEVIER
SAUNDERS

3251 Riverport Lane
St. Louis, Missouri 63043

STUDENT WORKBOOK FOR THE ADMINISTRATIVE DENTAL ASSISTANT   ISBN-13: 978-1-4377-1357-2
THIRD EDITION

Notices

Knowledge and best practice in this field are constantly changing. As new research and experience broaden our understanding, changes in research methods, professional practices, or medical treatment may become necessary.

Practitioners and researchers must always rely on their own experience and knowledge in evaluating and using any information, methods, compounds, or experiments described herein. In using such information or methods they should be mindful of their own safety and the safety of others, including parties for whom they have a professional responsibility.

With respect to any drug or pharmaceutical products identified, readers are advised to check the most current information provided (i) on procedures featured or (ii) by the manufacturer of each product to be administered, to verify the recommended dose or formula, the method and duration of administration, and contraindications. It is the responsibility of practitioners, relying on their own experience and knowledge of their patients, to make diagnoses, to determine dosages and the best treatment for each individual patient, and to take all appropriate safety precautions.

To the fullest extent of the law, neither the Publisher nor the authors, contributors, or editors, assume any liability for any injury and/or damage to persons or property as a matter of products liability, negligence or otherwise, or from any use or operation of any methods, products, instructions, or ideas contained in the material herein.

Vice President and Publisher: Linda Duncan
Executive Editor: John Dolan
Managing Editor: Kristin Hebberd
Developmental Editor: Joslyn Dumas
Publishing Services Managers: Julie Eddy and Hemamalini Rajendrababu
Project Managers: Marquita Parker and Srikumar Narayanan
Designer: Maggie Reid

Working together to grow
libraries in developing countries

www.elsevier.com | www.bookaid.org | www.sabre.org

ELSEVIER   BOOK AID International   Sabre Foundation

Printed in the United States of America

Last digit is print number: 9 8 7 6 5 4 3 2 1

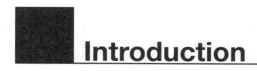

Introduction

TO THE STUDENT

The Student Workbook, DVD-ROM, and Evolve companion website have been designed to help you perfect the skills and objectives presented in *The Administrative Dental Assistant*, 3rd Edition. To help you achieve these objectives, this workbook includes the following features:

- An **Introduction** briefly states the key concept and goals of each chapter.
- **Learning Objectives** identify the concepts and skills that are necessary to master the goal of each chapter.
- **Exercises** ask questions that require you to list information, identify key concepts, and match terms with their definitions. Short-answer questions direct you to solve problems and sequence activities. These exercises are intended to help you achieve the objectives in the textbook by providing a means by which you can study, work with others, and develop necessary skills.
- **Activity Exercises** help you apply information learned to complete tasks that are similar to tasks you will encounter as an administrative dental assistant. The activities require you to use information assembled in one activity to complete the next task. It is very important that you complete the tasks in the order in which they are presented. Before moving on to the next task, you should verify the correctness of the completed task. Referring to information identified in the "Anatomy of..." figures and procedures outlined in the textbook may prove helpful. *Remember:* The tasks are sequenced and must be completed in the order presented.
- **Dentrix Exercises** introduce you to a *real-world* dental practice management software. Dentrix is a leader in dental practice management software and dental office technology integration. The DVD provided in this workbook is the Dentrix Learning Edition, which is a special version of Dentrix G4 designed specifically for educational purposes. It includes a preloaded database of patients and also offers users the ability to add patients of their own for practice. The accompanying *User's Guide* walks you through all the tasks and functions of the program.
- The companion Evolve website for *The Administrative Dental Assistant* was created specifically help enhance the experiences of both students and instructors using the textbook and workbook. Accessible via http://evolve.elsevier. com/Gaylor/ada, the following resources are provided:
  - Glossary Flashcards
  - Procedure Ordering Exercises
  - Image Identification Exercises
  - WebLinks

Plus...

"Day in the Life" Simulation Tool

The features of this interactive software are designed to guide you through simulated tasks typical to a dental business office. Each day of the week in the program increases in difficulty and introduces new concepts. Concepts are directly related to material in the textbook. Later days of the week will require you to independently apply information and concepts that you have learned in the textbook. You may find the exercises to have more significance after completing Chapters 3 through 17.

The interactive program simulates a "Day in the Life of an Administrative Dental Assistant" and challenges you to complete tasks as they would occur in the workplace, such as organizing functions, prioritizing tasks, solving problems, and completing daily tasks typical of an administrative dental assistant. Exam and study modes incorporated into the program provide flexibility in teaching and learning. Whereas the exam mode requires you to log in and complete the tasks in order from Monday through Friday, tracking your progress and outputting a results sheet, the study mode allows you to enter any day and time throughout the weeklong exercise to practice or review specific procedures.

- A variety of tasks typical in practice management software are included: entering and updating patient data, posting payment and treatment procedures, submitting insurance e-claims for payment, evaluating reports, and scheduling appointments.

- Patients arrive for appointments, and you must complete related tasks such as updating patient information and completing the checkout process. The mail arrives on a daily basis and must be processed. The telephone rings, and you must take care of the caller.
- Pop-ups ask you questions about a particular subject relevant to the task at hand. Prompts indicate whether you have answered the question correctly or incorrectly and provide a rationale. (You can go back and view the correct response if you have answered incorrectly.)

I hope that you will find the textbook and the accompanying material useful in pursuing an exciting career as a member of a dental healthcare team.

Linda J. Gaylor

Contents

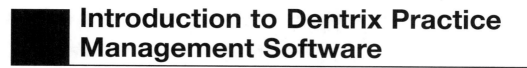

Introduction to Dentrix Practice Management Software

TIPS FOR A SUCCESSFUL INSTALLATION

These steps have been prepared to help minimize or eliminate any issues when installing the Dentrix Learning Edition. For a successful installation, follow the steps below exactly. Please read through all the steps before attempting to install the Learning Edition.

1. Ensure System Meets the System Requirements

For optimal performance with the Learning Edition, it is important to review the system requirements and make sure your system can accommodate them before you install the Learning Edition. The Dentrix Learning Edition system requirements are available at www.dentrix.com/training/dentrix-learning-edition.aspx.
Please be aware of the following:

- The Dentrix Learning Edition runs on a Windows platform and can run on only Microsoft Windows XP or higher.
- The computer's graphics card may need to be upgraded to take advantage of the 3-D modeling features in the Learning Edition.
- Adequate processor speed is important to help reduce or eliminate any latency/performance issues as they relate to the Learning Edition. The amount of free memory on the computer can greatly impact the performance of the computer and also the performance of the overall Dentrix system. Reducing or eliminating the number of unnecessary processes on a computer can significantly improve a computer's performance.

When the system requirements are closely scrutinized and adhered to, the potential for a successful installation experience increases dramatically.

2. Check Available Disk Space

From the Start menu, select My Computer and highlight the C: drive icon. Select View > Details from the menu bar, or right-click on the C: drive icon and select Properties. The Local Disk Properties dialog box appears. The General tab will display the Used and Free Disk Space.

Consult the Dentrix Learning Edition System Requirements to view the required free hard disk space for workstations. The current Dentrix system requirements are available online at www.dentrix.com/training/dentrix-learning-edition.aspx. You may experience slowness if your system does not meet the requirements for available memory or hard drive space. If your system is very deficient in memory, the Learning Edition might not be able to install on your system until you upgrade your system and get more memory.

3. IMPORTANT! Close All Other Applications

Look at the Windows Notification Area (normally in the bottom, right corner of the screen, near the system time) and close any programs that appear there. As with most programs, you must disable any antivirus software on the computer and the Windows screensaver for the duration of the installation. When the install is complete, enable the antivirus software and the Windows screensaver.

4. Follow the Installation Instructions

Follow the step-by-step instructions in this guide to install the Dentrix Learning Edition.

5. Finish the Installation Completely

Do not interrupt the installation process, even if it looks as though nothing is happening. You will be prompted when the installation is ready to continue. Terminating an installation prior to completion could affect the integrity of the database.

INSTALLING THE DENTRIX LEARNING EDITION

NOTE: If you are using Windows Vista, you may see messages during the installation process that are not shown in these steps. Follow the on-screen prompts for those messages as they appear and continue with the installation as directed in the steps below.

All Dentrix content within this section courtesy Henry Schein Practice Solutions, American Fork, Utah.

1. Insert the Dentrix Learning Edition DVD into the DVD drive. If the DVD drive is equipped with AutoStart technology, the **Dentrix G4 Install Welcome** screen appears within a few seconds (see below).
   - If you see the Welcome screen, proceed to step 2.
   - If the Welcome screen does not appear:

a. Click the Windows® **Start** button and select **Run**. The **Run** dialog box appears.

b. Type **D:Disk1Setup** in the command line (where D: is the drive letter for the DVD drive). Click the **OK** button to begin the installation.

c. Click **Install Software**. The screen that appears lists the products you can install. From this screen, you can install the Dentrix Learning Edition and the Required Components.

2. Click the **Install Required Components** install option to display the Required Components information (see below). Follow the instructions below to install the required components.

INSTALL
SOFTWARE   IMPORTANT
INSTALLATION TIPS   ADD-ON
PRODUCTS   CONTACT
US   CUSTOMER
SERVICE   EXPLORE
THIS CD

DENTRIX®

G4

INSPIRED

REQUIRED COMPONENTS

These components—.NET Framework, DirectX 9.0, Windows Journal Viewer, and Crystal Reports .NET Components are required for many of the new and exciting features of DENTRIX G4 to function properly. These components will be automatically installed when you install DENTRIX G4. Select "INSTALL NOW" to launch a customized install of these components.

INSTALL NOW

▸ INSTALL DENTRIX G4

▸ INSTALL DXMOBILE

▸ INSTALL REQUIRED COMPONENTS

EXIT

a. Click **Install Now** to install the required components. The InstallShield Wizard will perform a check of your system to verify that all the required components are installed. After the InstallShield Wizard has performed the check, a screen appears with a list of the required components and whether or not they are installed on your system (see following page).

NOTE: If you already have all the required components installed, click Finish to close the Required Components install dialog box and return to the main installation screen.

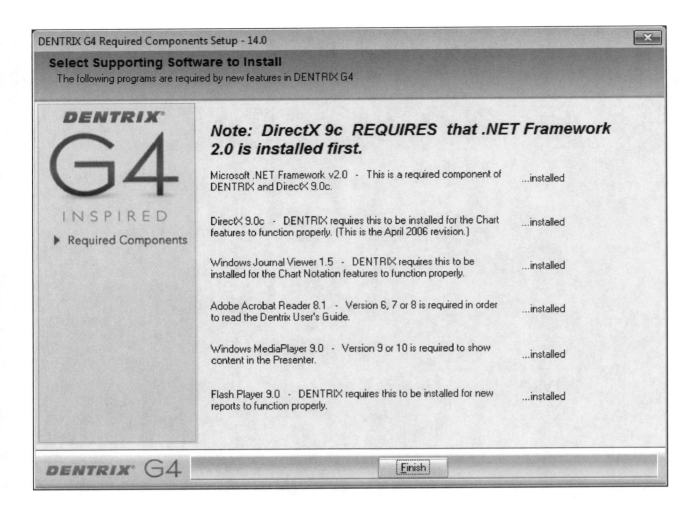

DENTRIX G4 Required Components Setup - 14.0

Select Supporting Software to Install
The following programs are required by new features in DENTRIX G4

DENTRIX G4
INSPIRED
▶ Required Components

Note: DirectX 9c REQUIRES that .NET Framework 2.0 is installed first.

Microsoft .NET Framework v2.0 - This is a required component of DENTRIX and DirectX 9.0c.   ...installed

DirectX 9.0c - DENTRIX requires this to be installed for the Chart features to function properly. (This is the April 2006 revision.)   ...installed

Windows Journal Viewer 1.5 - DENTRIX requires this to be installed for the Chart Notation features to function properly.   ...installed

Adobe Acrobat Reader 8.1 - Version 6, 7 or 8 is required in order to read the Dentrix User's Guide.   ...installed

Windows MediaPlayer 9.0 - Version 9 or 10 is required to show content in the Presenter.   ...installed

Flash Player 9.0 - DENTRIX requires this to be installed for new reports to function properly.   ...installed

DENTRIX G4   [Finish]

b. Click **Install All** to install all the required components. If desired, you can install each component one at a time by clicking Install next to the component, waiting for the install to finish, and clicking Install on the next component.

As components are installed, you might receive several on-screen messages or prompts. Follow the on-screen prompts to install the required components.

NOTE: If you are installing Adobe Flash Player 9, you may see an error message during the install. Click OK to the error message. If other components need to be installed, the installation continues.

c. Once all the required components have been installed, click the **Close** button (the red "X" button in the top, right corner). An **Exit Setup** message appears (see below).

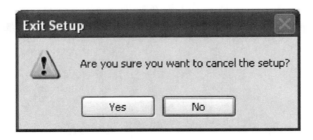

Exit Setup

⚠ Are you sure you want to cancel the setup?

[Yes]   [No]

d. Click **Yes** on the Exit Setup message to indicate that you want to cancel the setup and return to the Required Components information on the main install screen.

x

3. Click **Install Dentrix G4**. The **Dentrix Learning Edition installation information** appears (see below).

| INSTALL SOFTWARE | IMPORTANT INSTALLATION TIPS | ADD-ON PRODUCTS | CONTACT US | CUSTOMER SERVICE | EXPLORE THIS CD |

DENTRIX®
G4
INSPIRED

DENTRIX G4

To begin the installation of DENTRIX G4, click "INSTALL NOW" then sit back and watch as we add new features, tools, and functionality that transforms your DENTRIX system into a richer, more robust system. **Please refer to** "Important Installation Tips" before installing DENTRIX G4.

INSTALL NOW

▶ INSTALL DENTRIX G4

▶ INSTALL DXMOBILE

▶ INSTALL REQUIRED COMPONENTS

EXIT

Introduction to Dentrix Practice Management Software

4. Click the **Install Now** link at the bottom of the Dentrix Learning Edition installation information. The InstallShield Wizard loads and the **Welcome** screen appears (see below).

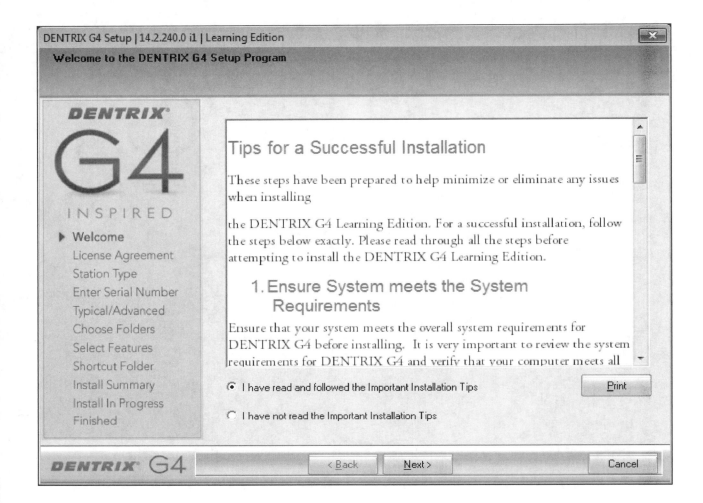

5. Read the Tips for a Successful Installation on this screen. When you have read the tips, mark **I have read and followed the tips for a successful installation** and click **Next** to continue. The **License Agreement** screen appears (see below).

   NOTE: If you want to print the Tips for a Successful Installation, click the Print button.

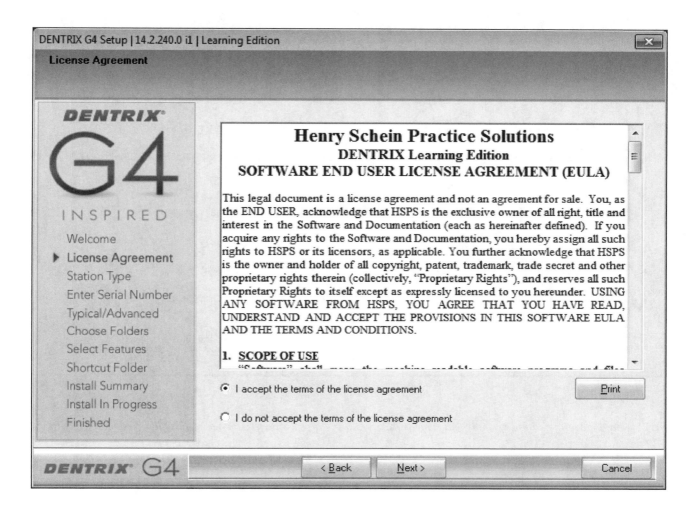

6. Read the Dentrix Learning Edition Software End User License Agreement. When you have read the document, mark **I accept the terms of the license agreement** and click **Next** to continue.

   NOTE: You can print a copy of the Dentrix Learning Edition Software End User License Agreement by clicking the Print button.

The InstallShield Wizard runs a System Requirements check. If your system meets the requirements, the Install continues to step 8. If your system does not meet the requirements, the **System Requirements Notice** dialog box appears and lists the deficiencies in your system (see below).

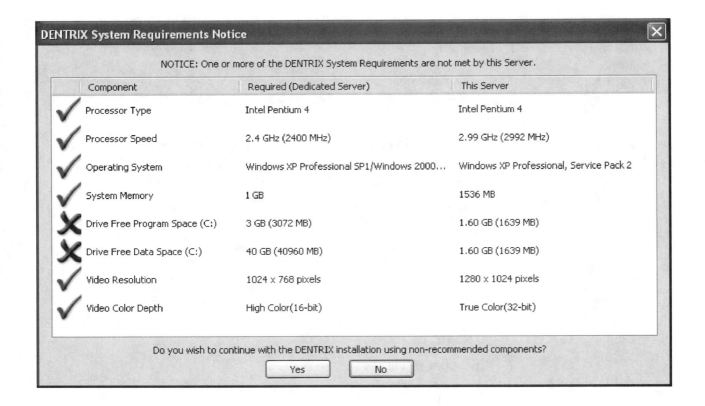

NOTE: The Learning Edition system requirements are available at www.dentrix.com/training/dentrix-learning-edition. aspx.

7. If the **System Requirements Notice** appears, verify the system requirements. A green check mark indicates that a component meets the requirements. A red "X" indicates that a component does not meet the requirements. Click **Yes** to continue the installation without meeting the recommended system requirements. The **Choose Folders** screen appears (see below).

If desired, you can click **No** to stop the installation and upgrade your system. However, that is not required for the Dentrix Learning Edition.

NOTE: The Dentrix Learning Edition may still function if your system does not meet the requirements. However, you may experience slowness if your system does not meet the requirements for available memory or hard drive space. If your system is very deficient in memory, the Learning Edition might not be able to install on your system until you upgrade your system and get more memory.

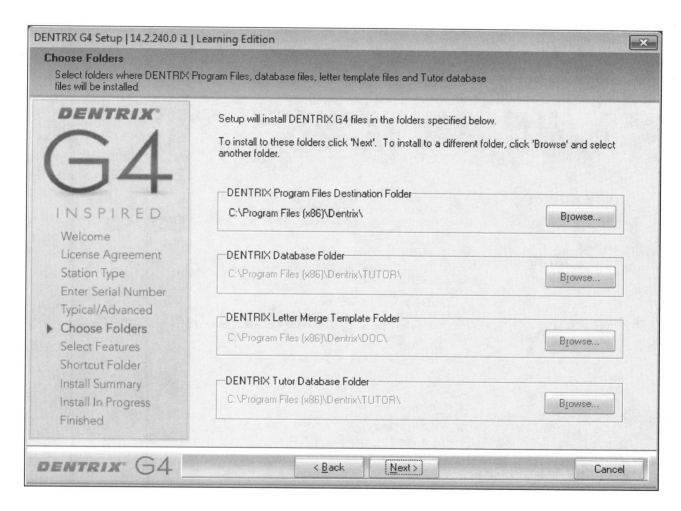

Introduction to Dentrix Practice Management Software

8. Select the folder where you want to store the Dentrix Learning Edition program files. If you do not want to store the program files in the folder that is recommended on the screen, you can select a new folder. Otherwise, leave the folder location as it is.

NOTE: The following folder locations are listed on the screen with the program files. With the Learning Edition, you can only change the location of the program files. The explanations below are for your reference only.

- *Program Files: The executable files that are required to make the program run. Your program files should be stored in the place where you want the Dentrix Learning Edition files to be stored.*
- *Database Files: The files that include your patient information files and the program settings that are specific to your office. The Tutor database is automatically set as your database.*
- *Letter Merge Templates: The Microsoft Word default letter templates that are used during the letter merge. These templates are automatically saved to the DOC folder.*
- *Tutor Database: A practice database that is used for training. These files are automatically installed.*

If you want to use the default folder location for the program files, click **Next**. If you want to change the program file folder location, click **Browse** and navigate to the desired location. The **Install Summary** screen appears (see below).

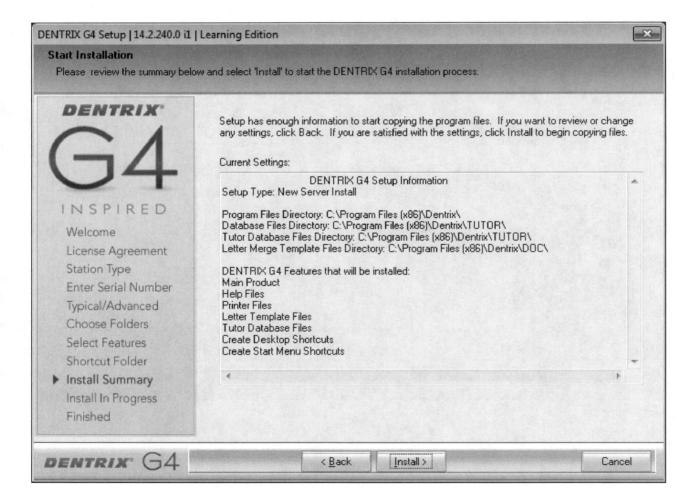

9. Click **Install** to begin installing the Dentrix Learning Edition. After a few minutes, the **Guru Limited Edition Server Installation Wizard** appears (see below).

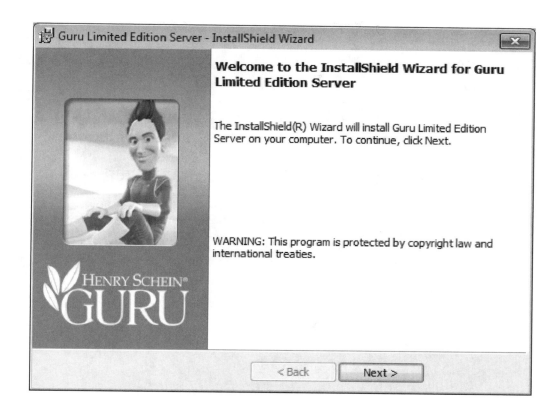

Introduction to Dentrix Practice Management Software

10. Guru Limited Edition is a patient education tool that can be accessed from the Dentrix Chart. Click **Next** on the **Guru Limited Edition Server Welcome** screen to continue with the installation. The **Guru Limited Edition license agreement** appears (see below).

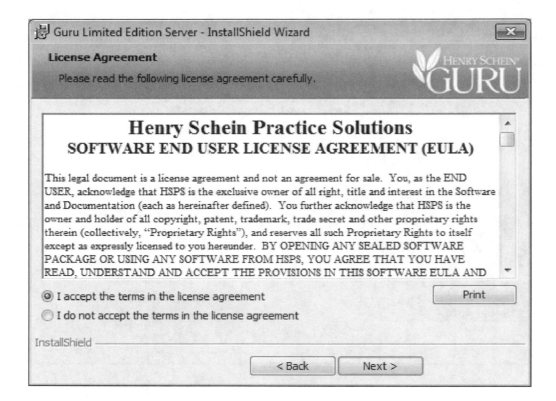

11. Read the Guru Limited Edition Software End User License Agreement. When you have read the document, mark **I accept the terms of the license agreement** and click **Next** to continue. The **Firewall Configuration** screen appears (see below).

NOTE: You can print a copy of the Guru Learning Edition Software End User License Agreement by clicking the Print button.

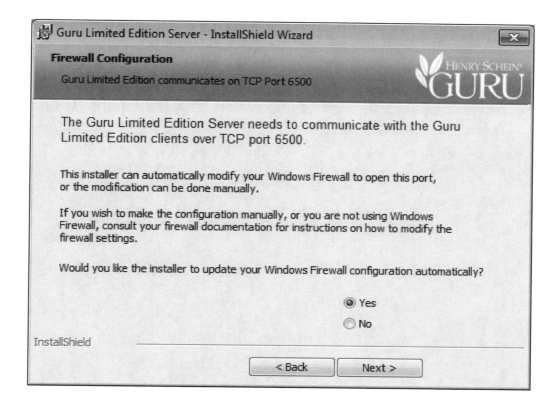

Introduction to Dentrix Practice Management Software

12. With the commercial edition of Dentrix, the Guru Limited Edition Server needs access to a specific port in the system to function properly. Typically, this port is blocked by firewall protection.

   With the Learning Edition, the Guru Limited Edition Server does not need to access this port, so you do not need to allow Guru to change your firewall configuration. Mark **No** on the **Firewall Configuration** screen. Click **Next** to continue with the installation. The **Ready to Install** screen appears (see below).

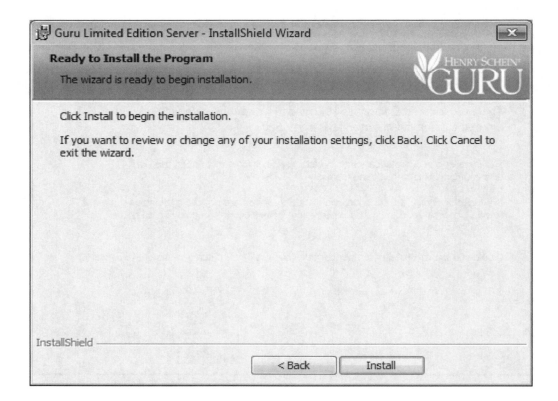

13. Click **Install** to begin the Guru Limited Edition Server installation. The **InstallShield Wizard Complete** screen appears when the install is finished (see below).

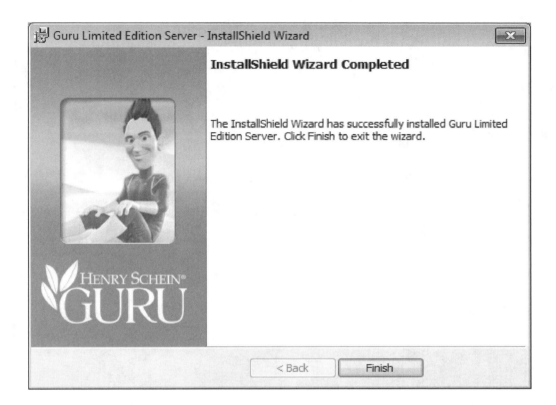

Introduction to Dentrix Practice Management Software

14. Click **Finish** to complete the Guru Limited Edition Server installation. The install continues with the rest of the Dentrix Learning Edition installation.

    After the Dentrix software has been installed, the **Setup Complete** screen appears (see below).

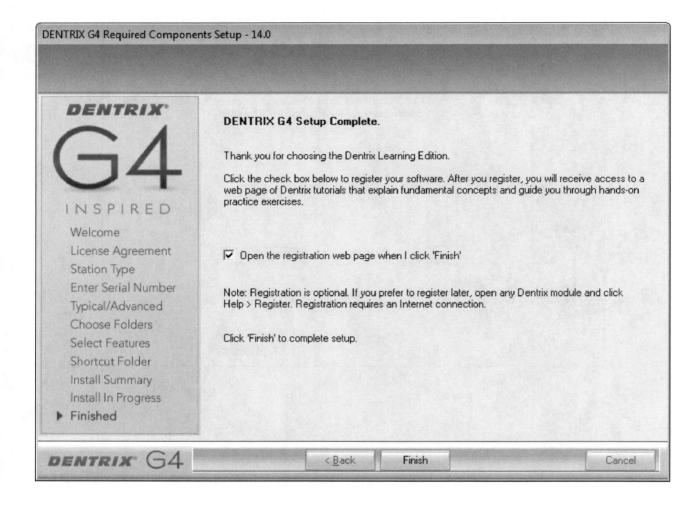

15. Click **Finish** to finish the Dentrix Learning Edition installation. The InstallShield Wizard will close and you will return to the **Dentrix Learning Edition installation** screen (see Figure i-5). If you checked the box to register the Dentrix Learning Edition, the registration page appears. See Registering the Dentrix Learning Edition section for more information about registering.

16. Click **Exit** to close the **Dentrix Learning Edition installation** screen. The InstallShield Wizard places six shortcuts on your Windows Desktop. These shortcuts open Dentrix modules and give you access to the Dentrix G4 User's Guide (see below).

- **Appointments**: Opens the Dentrix Appointment Book, the module you use to schedule patient appointments and manage your schedule.
- **Family File**: Opens the Dentrix Family File, the module you use to enter patient records and manage patient information.
- **Ledger**: Opens the Dentrix Ledger, the module you use to enter payments and manage accounts.
- **Office Manager**: Opens the Dentrix Office Manager, the module you use to run reports and set up practice defaults.
- **Patient Chart**: Opens the Dentrix Patient Chart, the module you use to chart treatment and enter clinical notes.
- **Dentrix Launcher:** Opens the Dentrix Launcher tool, which shows the Dentrix modules in the context of an office and helps you open the correct module for the task you want to perform.
- **Dentrix G4 User's Guide**: Opens a PDF of the Dentrix G4 User's Guide.
- **Productivity Pack 7 Update Guide**: Opens a PDF of the guide that describes the new features that were added to Dentrix G4 in Productivity Pack 7.
- **Productivity Pack 8 Update Guide**: Opens a PDF of the guide that describes the new features that were added to Dentrix G4 in Productivity Pack 8.

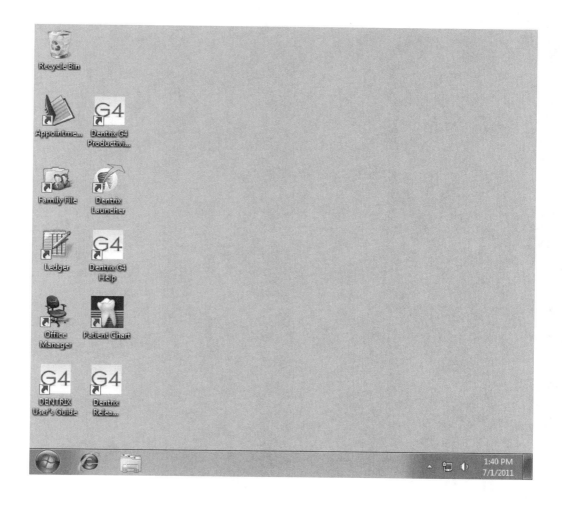

Introduction to Dentrix Practice Management Software

REGISTERING THE DENTRIX LEARNING EDITION

Registration is not required with the Dentrix Learning Edition. However, when you register you will receive access to a web page of Dentrix tutorials that explain fundamental concepts and guide you through hands-on practice exercises. For assistance with registration, please download the detailed Dentrix Learning Edition Installation Instructions available at www.dentrix.com.

If you do not register the Learning Edition during the installation, you can register at any time by clicking **Help > Register** in any Dentrix module.

NOTE: You must have an Internet connection and provide an email address in order to register the Learning Edition.

DISABLING THE ESYNC AND WEBSYNC

The eSync and WebSync are processes that run automatically with the commercial edition of Dentrix. You do not need to use these processes with the Dentrix Learning Edition. It is recommended that you disable these processes to prevent them from running automatically. Follow the instructions below to disable the eSync and WebSync.

Disabling the eSync

eSync is the process by which information is passed between the commercial edition of Dentrix and some of the Dentrix add-on features that are not available with the Learning Edition. It is important to disable this process and prevent it from running automatically with the Learning Edition.

NOTE: If you do not disable eSync, it will run automatically and you will receive eSync notifications daily. It is important to disable eSync to prevent it from running automatically.

The eSync setup is located in your computer's Notification Area. The eSync icon looks like a white 'e' in a red circle (see below).

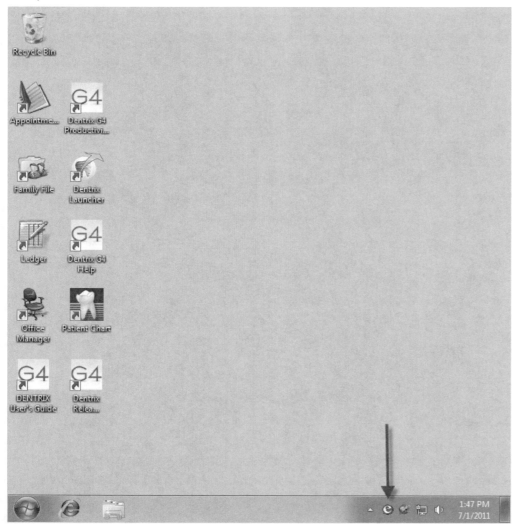

Follow the steps below to prevent the eSync from running automatically:

1. Locate the eSync icon in the Windows Notification Area. If the icon appears in the Notification Area, skip to step 2. If the icon does not appear in the Notification Area, follow steps a – b.
    a. Click the Windows **Start** button, select **All Programs**, and select **Startup** from the menu.
    b. Select **eSync Reminder** from the **Startup** menu. The **eSync** icon appears in the Notification Area.
2. Right-click the eSync icon and select **Open eSync Setup**. The **eSync Setup** dialog box appears (see below).

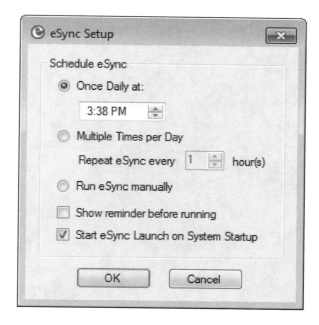

3. To prevent eSync from running automatically every day, mark **Run eSync Manually**. Do not change the other settings in the dialog box.
4. Click **OK** to the confirmation message that appears.
5. Click **OK** to close the **eSync Setup** dialog box. The eSync process is now disabled.

Disabling the WebSync

WebSync is the process through which information is transferred between Dentrix and eCentral with the commercial edition of Dentrix. It is important to disable this process and prevent it from running automatically with the Learning Edition.

NOTE: If you do not disable the WebSync, it will run automatically and you will receive WebSync notifications daily. It is important to disable the WebSync to prevent it from running automatically.

The WebSync Reminder icon is located in your Notification Area. The icon looks like a world with red and blue arrows around it (see below).

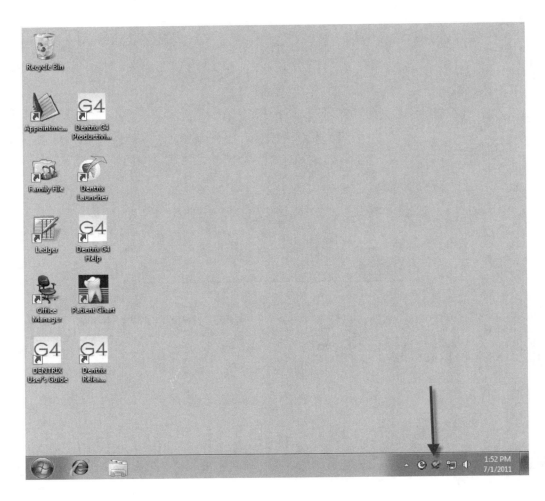

Follow the steps below to prevent WebSync from running automatically:

1. Locate the WebSync Reminder icon in the Notification Area. If the icon appears in the Notification Area, skip to step 2. If the icon does not appear in the Notification Area, follow steps a – b.
   a. Click the Windows **Start** button, select **All Programs**, and select **Startup** from the menu.
   b. Select **WebSync Reminder** from the **Startup** menu. The **WebSync Reminder** icon appears in the Notification Area.
2. Right-click the **WebSync Reminder** icon and select **Open the DXWeb Toolbar**. The **DXWeb Toolbar** appears (see below).

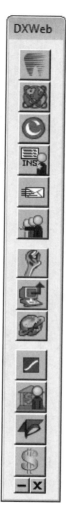

3. Click the **Settings** button (see below) and select **WebSync Wizard** from the menu.

4. Click **Next** on the **WebSync Wizard Welcome** screen (see below).

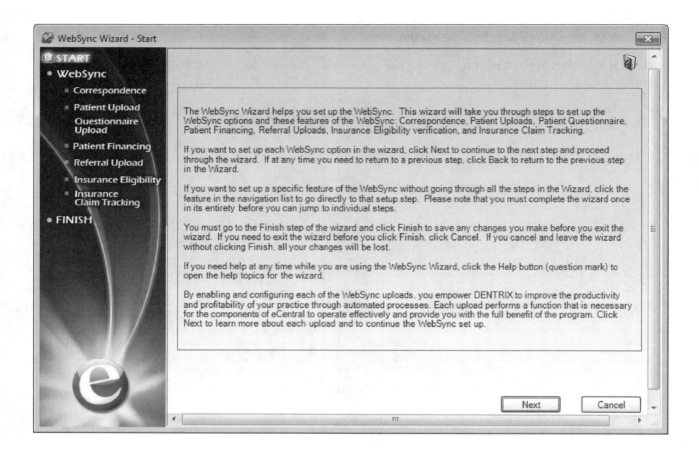

Introduction to Dentrix Practice Management Software

5. Mark **Do Not Run WebSync Automatically** in the Schedule Websync section of the **WebSync** screen (see below). Do not change the rest of the settings on the screen.

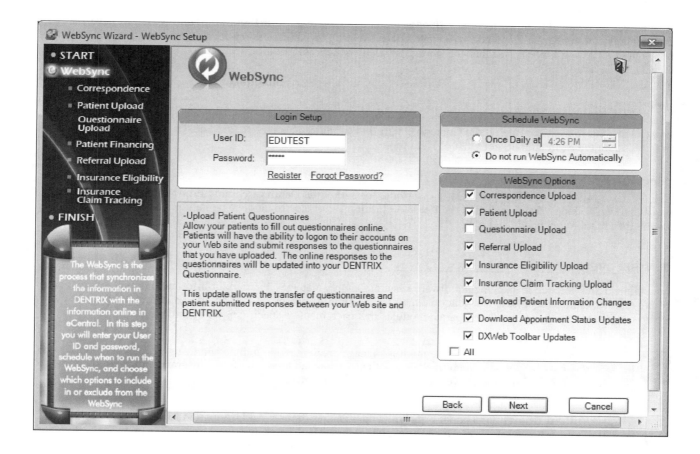

6. Click **Next** on each subsequent screen until you get to the end of the Wizard.
7. Click **Finish** to close the WebSync Wizard.
8. Click the small **"X"** in the bottom right, corner of the DXWeb Toolbar to close it.

Congratulations! You have installed and registered your copy of the Dentrix Learning Edition. If you need help, you can use any of the resources listed below.

On-Demand Training

Additional information, including on-demand software tutorials, can be found on the On-Demand Training web page. Our tutorials explain fundamental concepts and guide you through hands-on practice exercises. You can even check your understanding with simple quizzes.

To access on-demand training, from any Dentrix module, click **Help > On-Demand Training**. If you have an Internet connection, the On-Demand Login page opens. Before you can access on-demand training, you must register the Dentrix Learning Edition. See the Registering the Dentrix Learning Edition section in this guide for instructions to register the Learning Edition.

Help Files

To access the Help files, open any module and click Help > Contents. The Dentrix Help window appears. In the Help, you can use the navigation Tree on the Contents tab to find a feature in a specific module. Or, you can type key words in the filed on the Search tab to get a list of Help topics.

User's Guide

The Dentrix G4 User's Guide is provided in electronic format on the Dentrix Learning Edition DVD and is saved on the Windows Desktop when you install the Learning Edition. With electronic documentation, you can quickly search for the information you need.

DENTRIX OVERVIEW

As a clinical and practice management software system, Dentrix manages a variety of information, including patient demographics, clinical details, and production analysis. To simplify the process of entering and finding data, the Dentrix software is divided into five separate modules that each manage specific types of information.

 Family File: The Family File module manages patient demographic and insurance information. From this module you will keep track of a patient's name, address, employer, insurance information, notes, and continuing care, as well as other important information.

 Patient Chart: The Patient Chart module manages the clinical information for patients. The Patient Chart is a powerful, yet easy-to-use, application. The Chart allows you to post existing, completed, and recommended procedures using common textbook symbols. Additionally, the Chart helps users keep extensive and detailed notes regarding patient care.

Several sub-modules of the Chart help users manage other clinical functions. The Presenter is a unique case presentation program that displays the treatment plan costs in terms of primary and secondary insurance portions and the estimated patient portion. The Perio Chart is an unparalleled periodontal data maintenance tool.

 Ledger: Patient accounts are managed in the Ledger. Because Dentrix is a seamlessly integrated system, procedures completed in the Patient Chart are automatically posted in the Ledger. All financial transactions are recorded in the Ledger, including charges, payments, and adjustments. The Ledger provides information concerning patient portion versus insurance portion, deductibles owed, and payment arrangements.

 Office Manager: The Office Manager offers useful, customizable reports including day sheets, aging reports, financial reports, patient lists, reference reports, and more.

Additionally, the Office Manager integrates with Microsoft Word to create effective, professional-looking letters that are available at the click of a mouse. These letters include welcome letters, congratulatory letters, thank you letters, and a variety of appointment and continuing care (recall) reminders, progress reports, and collection notices. The Office Manager contains a set of utilities and commands that make customizing Dentrix easy.

Appointment Book: Managing appointments has never been easier than with the Dentrix Appointment Book. The Appointment Book offers all the functionality of the Appointment List in a user-friendly graphical interface. The Appointment Book offers goal-oriented scheduling with the flexibility to make one-time changes. Appointment Book's convenient toolbars and Flip Tabs make navigating through the Appointment Book, searching for open times, and organizing appointments simple and quick. With the click of a button, the Appointment Book allows you to schedule appointments, record broken appointments, print route slips, and dial a patient's phone number directly from the computer. And, like the standard Dentrix modules, the Appointment Book provides access to other Dentrix modules from the toolbar.

Important Buttons to Know

 Patient Chart: This button appears on every major toolbar throughout Dentrix except within the Patient Chart module. Click this button to open and display the current patient's chart.

 Family File: This button appears on every major toolbar throughout Dentrix except within the Family File. Click this button to open and display the current patient's family file.

 Ledger: This button appears on every major toolbar throughout Dentrix except within the Ledger. Click this button to open and display the current patient's ledger.

 Appointments: This button appears on every major toolbar throughout Dentrix except within the Appointment Book or Appointment List. Click this button to open the Appointment Book (if installed) or the Appointment List to the current date (the current system date).

 Office Manager: This button appears on every major toolbar throughout Dentrix except within the Office Manager. Click this button to open the Office Manager.

 Select Patient: This button appears on every major toolbar throughout Dentrix except within the Office Manager and the Appointment Book. Click this button to select a patient from the patient database.

 Quick Letters: This button appears on every major toolbar throughout Dentrix except within the Office Manager. Click this button to print pre-written letters concerning a patient's account or clinical diagnosis and treatment plan.

 Continuing Care (Recall): This button appears on every major toolbar throughout Dentrix except within the Office Manager. Click this button to view recall appointments assigned to a patient and track whether or not an appointment has been made.

 Office Journal: This button appears on every major toolbar throughout Dentrix except within the Office Journal. Office Journal acts as a contact manager for your dental office. All correspondence and contacts made with patients can be tracked and recorded by clicking the Office Journal button.

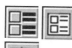 **Questionnaires:** This button appears on every major toolbar throughout Dentrix except within the Office Manager. Click this button to open the Questionnaires module from which you can view questionnaires, enter questionnaire responses, sign questionnaires, and update the Family File with information provided through questionnaire responses. The Questionnaires button looks like a blank form when the selected patient does not have any questionnaire responses attached. The Questionnaires button looks like a form with a red check mark when the patient has questionnaire responses attached.

 Prescriptions: This button appears on every major toolbar throughout Dentrix except within the Office Manager. Click this button to open a window from which prescriptions can be printed and a notation that a drug has been prescribed can be made.

 Medical Alerts: This button appears on the Family File, Patient Chart, and Presenter toolbars. The button is red when a patient has a health condition requiring attention. Click this button to open a list of a patient's medical alerts. Medical alerts can be added, edited, or deleted from this list.

Patient Picture: This button appears on all modules except within the Ledger and Office Manager. Click this button to open a digital photograph of the selected patient. If no picture is assigned to the patient, the icon will be a graphic of a framed photo. If a picture is assigned to the patient, the icon will be a miniature of that picture.

  Patient Alerts: This button appears on every major toolbar throughout Dentrix except within the Office Manager. Click this button to add or edit Patient Alerts for the selected patient.

  Document Center: This button appears on every major toolbar throughout Dentrix except within the Document Center. Click this button to open the Document Center window in which documents can be viewed, edited, and attached to patients, providers, employers, referrals, and insurance carriers. The Document Center icon looks like a closed filing cabinet if the selected patient does not have documents attached in the Document Center module. The Document Center icon looks like a filing cabinet with paper in the open drawer if the selected patient has documents attached in the Document Center module.

  Patient Referrals: This button appears on every major toolbar throughout Dentrix except within the Office Manager. Click this button to open a window in which patient referral information can be viewed, added, or edited.

 Treatment Planner: This button only appears in the Patient Chart module. Click this button to create new treatment plan cases, sign treatment consent forms, and view treatment case totals. The Treatment Planner button appears green when a treatment plan is saved for the selected patient.

 Presenter: This button only appears in the Patient Chart module. Click this button to present treatment case information and view patient education.

  Perio: This button only appears in the Patient Chart module. Click this button to chart perio scores, enter oral health data, and compare current oral health to previous exams. The Perio button has a blue background when a perio exam has been saved for the selected patient.

 Guru: This button only appears in the Patient Chart module. Click this button to launch Guru Limited Edition or Henry Schein Guru (if you have the full version installed) where you can view patient education topics, create patient education playlists, and create custom patient education topics.

USER SUPPORT

For technical support regarding the **installation** of Dentrix Learning Edition, first refer to the *Dentrix G4 User's Guide* found on the DVD-ROM. Further **installation support** is available by contacting Dentrix directly via phone at 1-800-DENTRIX (336-8749) or via email at *support@dentrix.com*. Further support information and options can be accessed at *www.dentrix.com/support/contact-us.aspx*. Questions about the exercises or functionality of the program should be directed to your instructor.

1 Orientation to the Dental Profession

INTRODUCTION

The dental profession of the twenty-first century will be a complex healthcare delivery system. As a member of the dental healthcare team, it is important that you understand the role of the dental assistant in all phases of the dental practice and the daily business operations. Those who will excel and become vital members of the dental healthcare team will have mastered multiple skills, will be flexible, and will work well in a team environment.

LEARNING OBJECTIVES

1. List the different traits of an effective dental administrative assistant.
2. Describe the many roles of the administrative dental assistant: office manager, business manager, receptionist, insurance biller, records manager, data processor, bookkeeper, and appointment scheduler.
3. Name the various members of the dental healthcare team and discuss the roles they play in the delivery of dental care.
4. Identify the rules and function of the Health Insurance Portability and Accountability Act of 1996, Administrative Simplification, as it applies to the dental healthcare system.
5. Examine the American Dental Association's *Principles of Ethics and Code of Professional Conduct,* and demonstrate an understanding of the content by explaining, discussing, and applying the principles.

EXERCISES

1. List the personal traits of an effective administrative dental assistant.

   _____

   _____

   _____

   _____

   _____

2. Refer to the traits you listed in Question No. 1, and select your strongest (or weakest) trait. Based on your selection, write a short paragraph (give an example) to support your selection.

   _____

   _____

   _____

   _____

   _____

3. List the responsibilities of a dental receptionist.

_____

_____

_____

_____

_____

4. List the duties of a records manager.

_____

_____

_____

_____

5. Match the following job description with the appropriate administrative assistant:

   a. _____ Typically will organize and oversee the daily operations of the office staff.

   b. _____ Manages the fiscal operation of the dental practice, develops marketing campaigns, negotiates contracts, and oversees the compliance of insurance programs.

   c. _____ Maintains all aspects of the patient's clinical chart according to preset standards.

   d. _____ Responsible for entering data into the computer system.

   e. _____ Organizes and maintains the daily schedule of patients.

A. Business Manager
B. Appointment Scheduler
C. Data Processor
D. Records Manager
E. Bookkeeper
F. Office Manager
G. Insurance Biller

In the following scenarios, it will be the responsibility of the administrative dental assistant to refer the patient to a specialist. In the blank, identify the specialist to whom you will refer the patient for treatment.

6. Mrs. Tracy has been diagnosed with periodontal disease. Dr. Edwards instructs you to refer her to Dr. Usher for a

consultation. Dr. Usher is a _____.

7. David Collins is a 4-year-old child with extensive dental caries. His mother has asked for the name of a dentist

who specializes in the treatment of children. You will refer David to a _____.

8. Chris Salinas has been given the diagnosis of four impacted wisdom teeth. Dr. Edwards instructs you to refer

Chris to an _____.

9. Judy Johnson was scheduled for an emergency visit. She has a tooth that is badly decayed. After Dr. Bradley examines Judy, he concludes that she will need a root canal. Judy will be referred to an _____.

10. Mr. Kelly is an 85-year-old man who has been wearing dentures for a number of years. Because of extensive alveolar bone loss on the mandibular arch, Dr. Edwards would like Mr. Kelly to see a _____ because of the complexity of the case.

11. Sally Davis is a 13-year-old young lady with very crowded teeth. Dr. Edwards requested a referral to an _____ for a consultation.

12. Mrs. Gonzales was scheduled for a biopsy of oral tissue. The biopsy was sent to an _____ for evaluation.

13. Dr. Parker is the director and chief dentist in a government-sponsored inner city dental clinic. The specialty Dr. Parker practices is _____.

14. Based on what you learned in this chapter, what do the following acronyms stand for?

    D.D.S. _____

    D.M.D. _____

    OSHA _____

    ADA _____

    CDA _____

    ADAA _____

    DANB _____

15. List and briefly describe the five principles of ethics identified by the ADA.

    _____

    _____

    _____

    _____

    _____

    _____

16. Define the following terms:

    Ethics:

    _____

    _____

Legal Standards:

_____

_____

Dental Practice Act:

_____

_____

17. What is the primary purpose of the Administrative Simplification provision of the HIPAA document?

18. List the four sets of HIPAA standandards and give a brief description of each standard.

1.

2.

3.

4.

DENTRIX EXERCISE*

Before you can begin this exercise it will be necessary to download the Dentrix G4 Learning Edition to your computer. Please review the instructions in the front of the workbook. You will also need to become familiar with the icons used to open various elements of the program such as Office Manager, Patient Chart, Family File, Appointments, Ledger, and the Dentrix *User's Guide.*

Practice Setup
With Dentrix, a default practice is set up for you in the Tutor database. You will be able to view and change some but not all of the information. When you attempt to edit information that is unchangeable, you will get an error notice. Click **OK** to close the message.

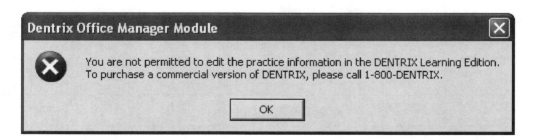

* Dentrix exercises based on content and screen captures courtesy Henry Schein Practice Solutions, American Fork, Utah.

Provider and Staff Setup

To view the practice information, in the Office Manager (open the Office Manager icon), select **Maintenance – Practice Setup – Practice Resource Setup.** The Practice Resource Setup dialog box appears.

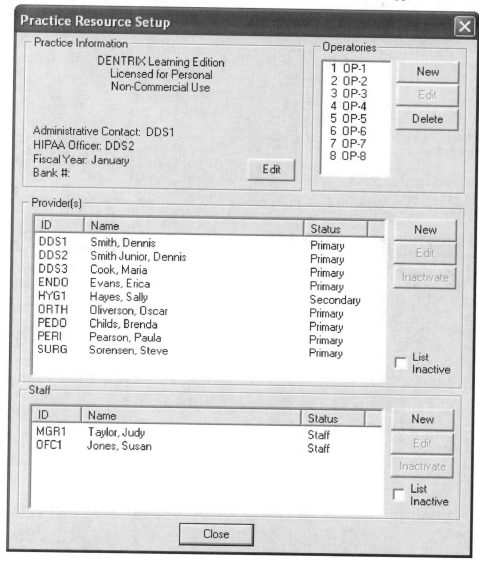

Answer the following questions with the information located in the **Practice Resource Setup** dialog box:

1. Who is the Administrative Contact (name)?

2. What dental specialty does Dr. Brenda Childs practice?

3. If a patient needed to be scheduled for a root canal, which provider would you select?

4. Who is the office manager?

Click **Close.**

Please note: With the commercial edition of Dentrix, you will have the ability to set up and edit practice information, providers, and staff members. For information on how to set up a practice, consult the Dentrix *User's Guide*, which is provided in electronic format on the Dentrix Learning Edition DVD and also saved on the Windows desktop when the Learning Edition is installed.

Operatory Setup

To add a new operatory:

1. In the Office Manager, select **Maintenance – Practice Setup – Practice Resource Setup**. The Practice Resource Setup dialog box appears (see above).

2. In the Operatories group box, click **New.**

3. Enter an ID for the operatory in the **ID** field (enter the first four letters of your name). This information will appear as an operatory in the appointment book.

4. Enter a description (use your name).

5. Click **Close.**

Procedure Codes Setup

You can set up new procedure codes to fit the needs of your office. The Learning Edition does not include the standard CDT codes. Because of copyright reasons, they have been replaced with non-ADA codes.

1. In the Office Manager, select **Maintenance – Practice Setup – Procedure Code Setup.** The Procedure Code Setup dialog box appears.

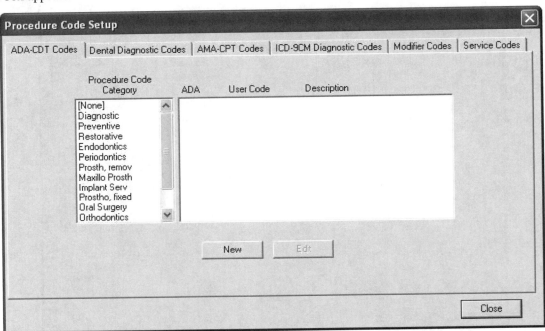

2. Click the **ADA-CDT Codes**, select Preventive, and scroll through the Procedure Code Category **Preventive** until you locate **X2397**.

3. Click **Edit**.

Answer the following questions:

1. What is the name of the dialog box?

2. What is the *Description?*

3. What is the fee charged BC/BS?

4. Edit the fee for Aetna to $54.00.

Click **Save** and **Close.**

6

Fee Schedule Setup

The Automatic Fee Schedule Changes utility allows you to change an entire fee schedule rather than changing one fee at a time. To use the Automatic Fee Schedule Changes utility

1. In the Office Manager, select **Maintenance – Practice Setup – Auto Fee Schedule Changes.** The Automatic Fee Schedule Changes dialog box appears:

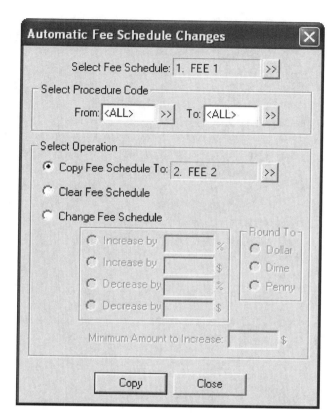

2. In *Select Operation,* click – **Change Fee Schedule.**

3. Increase the fees by 8%.

4. Click – **Change**.

5. Scroll to procedure code X1772 and click on it to select.

   Answer the following questions:

   ■ What was the *Fee #1 Office?*

   ■ What is the new fee?

6. Click **Edit**.

7. Change the fee to $130.00.

8. Click to save (**check mark**).

9. Click **Accept**.

10. Click **Close**.

To review all the setup features in detail refer to the Dentrix *User's Guide.*

Search for the **BOLDFACE CAPITALIZED** words seen in the list below in this word search puzzle.

Dental Healthcare Team Members

```
K N O I T C N U F D E D N A P X E D R C
E R N T A L H E A L T H C A R E T E E H
G A E B U S I N E S S M A N A G E R G A
M N M L E T I M B E R S T O G V L T A I
H S I W C I N N X M A Y E P B S J S N R
N Y Q T D T S A S B I G C W E Z A I A S
G S B L A B N X T U V J S Z R D Z N M I
U J B H O L F E M S R N S J M B T E E D
J V S X Y H U G M Z I A S I V A O I C E
N G R H M D C C C T F S N Q R G H G I E
Y U T Q G J D N R R N I S C A N R Y F O
N X C T T Y Z O M I S I S A E Z P H F F
A Z H L P R E D W T C X O R L S L V O T
G N D G Q Y O F R F Z O H P Y A E I H F
G D N O M G G A I D L I I X P J T C E E
T S I N O I T P E C E R M J B A D N P A
P R A C T I C E M A N A G E M E N T E N
S L V L V R E C O R D S M A N A G E R D
R E P E E K K O O B C S I J F X M B W Y
N S C C V X Q M A L O A L K L O M G G K
```

ADMINISTRATIVE Dental Assistant

APPOINTMENT Scheduler

BOOKKEEPER

BUSINESS MANAGER

Certified **DENTAL ASSISTANT**

CHAIRSIDE Dental Assistant

CIRCULATING (Roving) Assistant

Dental **HYGIENIST**

EXPANDED (Extended) **FUNCTION** Assistant

INSURANCE Biller

OFFICE MANAGER

Certified Dental **PRACTICE MANAGEMENT** Assistant

RECEPTIONIST

RECORDS MANAGER

2 Dental Basics

INTRODUCTION

The development of a professional dental vocabulary is essential for communicating with others. If you are unable to understand the dental language, it will be very difficult for you to carry out the fundamental duties of your job, such as appointment scheduling, insurance coding, clinical chart management, and billing.

LEARNING OBJECTIVES

1. List and describe the different areas of a dental office.
2. List the basic structures of the face and oral cavity.
3. Name the basic anatomical structures and tissues of the teeth.
4. Distinguish between different tooth numbering systems.
5. Interpret dental charting symbols.
6. Categorize basic dental procedures.
7. List basic chairside dental assisting duties and identify Occupational Safety and Health Administration and state regulations.

EXERCISES

1. Identify the different areas of the dental practice.

   a. _____ The first area to be viewed by the patient.

   b. _____ Area used by administrative dental assistants to perform daily business tasks.

   c. _____ A private area used to discuss confidential information with a patient.

   d. _____ Area where duties pertaining to the fiscal operation of the dental practice take place.

   e. _____ Area where patients are treated by the dentist, dental hygienist, and dental assistant.

   f. _____ Consists of a contaminated area and a clean area.

   g. _____ Dental x-rays are taken in this area.

   h. _____ Dental radiographic film is processed in this area.

   A. Sterilization area
   B. Clinical area
   C. Reception area
   D. Business office
   E. Nonclinical areas
   F. Staff room
   G. Darkroom
   H. Treatment rooms
   I. Consultation area
   J. Radiology room
   K. Storage area

2. Label the following diagram:

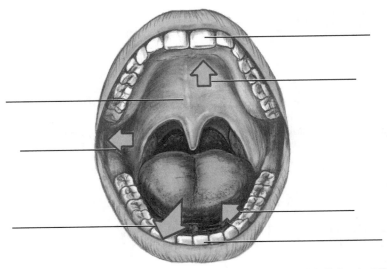

(From Fehrenbach MJ, Herring SW: *Illustrated anatomy of the head and neck,* ed 3, St Louis, 2007, Saunders.)

3. Label the following diagram:

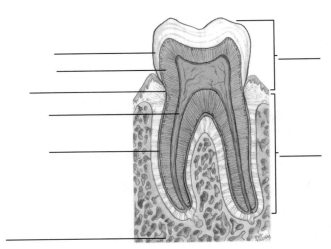

(From Bath-Balogh M, Fehrenbach MJ: *Illustrated dental embryology, histology, and anatomy,* ed 3, St Louis, 2011, Saunders.)

Using the patient chart below, complete the following tasks:

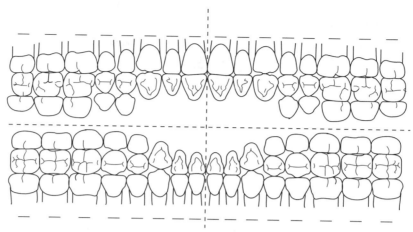

(From Bird DL, Robinson DS: *Modern dental assisting,* ed 10, St Louis, 2012, Saunders.)

4. Correctly number the teeth on the chart (space provided on the chart above the maxillary arch and below the mandibular arch) using the Universal Numbering System.

5. Correctly chart the following conditions using the symbols described in Chapter 2 (use red and blue pencil):

   a. Maxillary right third molar, impacted

   b. Maxillary right second molar, MO restoration

   c. Maxillary right second premolar, MOD caries

   d. Maxillary right central, bonded veneer

   e. Maxillary left central, bonded veneer

   f. Maxillary left first molar, DO restoration

   g. Maxillary left third molar, missing

   h. Mandibular left third molar, missing

   i. Mandibular left first molar, full gold crown

   j. Mandibular left cuspid, periapical abscess

   k. Mandibular right lateral, mesial composite

   l. Mandibular right second premolar, occlusal caries

   m. Mandibular right first molar, completed endodontic treatment, post and core, PFM

   n. Mandibular right third molar, needs to be extracted

DENTRIX EXERCISE (OPTIONAL)

Read the chapter entitled "Patient Chart" in the Dentrix *User's Guide.* (*Note*: The *User's Guide* is provided in electronic format on the Dentrix Learning Edition DVD and also saved on the Windows desktop when the Learning Edition is installed.) The Dentrix Patient Chart is a method of record keeping that incorporates four separate parts: (1) the Patient Chart, (2) the Perio Chart, (3) the Clinical Notes, and (4) the Treatment Planner.

For added practice, set up the Patient Chart according to the process outlined in the *User's Guide.* Select a patient who is already in the database and record the conditions outlined above in Question #5.

Chapter **2** **Dental Basics**

Unscramble each of the clue words. Copy the letters in the numbered cells into the cells with the same number below the scrambled words. Solve the phrase at the bottom.

Dental Procedures

MAAMGLA

```
                                              18
```

REBDIG

```
27   9          15
```

CATS SONRCW

```
29  11
```

WONRC

```
22      16
```

DENLAT PAYRIPOLXHS

```
28    4         1         20
```

NYALI

```
8
```

NOLAY

```
19
```

LICPOANER SUFDE TO TMLAE

```
3          13       14
```

BEAMEROVL PIRLATA

```
24                17
```

SIENR

```
10
```

SATREIVORTE TYISEDNRT

```
6         25
```

ORTO CALNA

```
23    2
```

SASTALNE

```
7
```

CALSUIRG STCONXIARET

```
26  21                        5
```

NEREEV CONSWR

```
12
```

```
 1  2  3  4  5  6  7    8  9 10 11   12 13   14 15 16 17 18 19   20 21 22 23 24 25 26 27 28 29
```

3 Communication Skills: Telephone Techniques

Communication is a two-way process by which information is transferred and shared between a sender and a receiver. It is important for the dental healthcare team to understand and practice effective communication skills.

LEARNING OBJECTIVES

1. Identify the five elements of the communications process.
2. Differentiate between verbal and nonverbal messages and describe how the two are used to send and receive messages.
3. Demonstrate how the dental healthcare team sends nonverbal cues.
4. Categorize the different types of interpersonal communication and describe how they are used in the dental profession.
5. Discuss the barriers to effective communication and express how members of the dental healthcare team can remove these barriers.
6. List the responsibilities of the sender that contribute to effective communication and list the responsibilities of the receiver in effective communication.
7. Identify and describe professional telephone manners.

EXERCISES

1. List the elements of the communication process that are linked together to complete the exchange of information.

_____

_____

_____

_____

_____

_____

_____

_____

2. Verbal messages can be divided into two categories. Name each category and give two examples.

- (Category) _____

   Example: _____

   _____

   Example: _____

   _____

- (Category) _____

    Example: _____

    _____

    Example: _____

    _____

3. What positive nonverbal messages can be sent from a member of the dental healthcare team to the patient? List the three examples given in the textbook.

    Example: _____

    Example: _____

    Example: _____

4. Interpersonal communication takes place when the sender and the receiver are exchanging information in real time. Match the type of transfer (typical to a dental practice) with the following statements:

    a. _____ Administrative assistant is instructed to call the pharmacy.

    b. _____ Patient calls to schedule an appointment for her children.

    c. _____ Hygienist gives oral hygiene instructions to a patient.

    d. _____ Office staff meeting is held.

    e. _____ Administrative assistant schedules patient's appointment.

    f. _____ Patient has a question concerning her statement.

    g. _____ Patient inquires about the types of dental insurance accepted.

    h. _____ Dentist consults with a specialist concerning the diagnosis and treatment plan of a patient.

    i. _____ Administrative assistant reviews financial arrangements with a patient.

    j. _____ Employee is given performance review.

    A. Patient to Dental Healthcare Team
    B. Dental Healthcare Team to Patient
    C. Team Member to Team Member
    D. Professional to Professional

5. Identify the type of barrier to effective communication that may take place in the following situations:

    a. _____ "Mr. Franklin, you are scheduled for a filling." (administrative assistant)

    b. _____ "I am not sure, but I think you should feel all right when the doctor is finished today." (administrative assistant)

    c. _____ "I don't understand why the dentist wants to fix a baby tooth." (parent)

    d. _____ "I don't think you will want to have the treatment if your insurance company does not pay." (administrative assistant)

6. When creating a positive telephone voice, it is important that you _____ .
   a. develop an active script
   b. smile
   c. learn new phrases
   d. all of the above

7. A telephone should be answered within _____ rings.
   a. 2
   b. 3
   c. 4
   d. 5

8. When you are answering the telephone, your greeting should include all of the following except
   a. identify the practice by name
   b. identify yourself by name
   c. use good listening skills
   d. time of day, for example, good morning, good afternoon

9. Personal telephone calls are appropriate when
   a. you personally answer the telephone
   b. you are not busy
   c. you ask the dentist first
   d. you have an emergency

10. The HIPAA Privacy Rule states that you must take appropriate and reasonable steps to keep a patient's personal health information private. Please describe how you would do this in a dental office.

_____

_____

_____

WHAT WOULD YOU DO?

Dr. Edwards informs you that her next study group will be holding an online video meeting. This is a new experience for both of you. You are tasked with researching the process and identifying what additional equipment (if any) you will need.

Hint: Do an Internet search on "types of video conferencing."

Using the clues below, fill in the crossword puzzle.

Elements of Communication

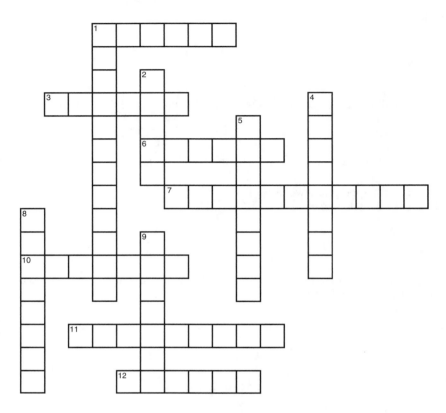

Across

1. Person who shares message
3. Specialized or technical terms
6. Communicate positive thoughts
7. State of believing
10. Format used for translating the message
11. Changes in the meaning of a word
12. Format used for translating the message

Down

1. Assumptions made on nonfactual information
2. An item that hinders communication
4. State of feeling
5. Reaction to the message
8. Person who receives the message
9. Translation of the idea

4 Written Correspondence

INTRODUCTION

Written communication includes different types of media and can be used to achieve a variety of objectives. Letters are used to communicate between patients, professionals, and employees. Written communications may be provided in the form of letters, newsletters, office manuals, and marketing strategies. In addition to creating effective correspondence, it is necessary to know how to process incoming and outgoing mail.

LEARNING OBJECTIVES

1. Discuss the four elements of letter writing style and compose a letter.
2. Describe letter style appearance as it applies to a finished business letter.
3. Recognize the different parts of a business letter.
4. Evaluate a completed business letter by identifying letter style format, judging letter style appearance, and assessing letter writing style.
5. Identify when HIPAA Privacy and Security Rules apply to written communications.
6. Discuss the various types of mail and determine how each type should be handled.

EXERCISES

Define the following letter writing elements of style:

Tone: _____

_____

_____

_____

Outlook: _____

_____

_____

_____

"You" technique: _____

_____

_____

_____

Organization: _____

_____

_____

_____

2. Compose one or two sentences that are examples of

Tone: _____

_____

_____

_____

Outlook: _____

_____

_____

_____

"You" technique: _____

_____

_____

_____

3. Match each of the following statements with the correct title:

a. _____ Address of the party receiving the letter.

b. _____ Alert the reader that there is more to the letter.

c. _____ Describes what the next step or expected outcome will be.

d. _____ Draws attention to the person you wish to read the letter.

e. _____ Draws attention to the subject of the correspondence.

f. _____ Final closing of the letter and is a courtesy.

g. _____ First paragraph and states the reason you are writing.

A. Subject line
B. Signer's identification
C. Salutation
D. Reference initials
E. Main body
F. Line spacing
G. Letterhead
H. Introduction
I. Inside address
J. Enclosure reminder
K. Dateline
L. Copy notation
M. Complimentary closing

h. _____ Gives details of the points that you stated in the introduction.

i. _____ Greeting.

j. _____ Identifies the dental practice that is sending the letter.

k. _____ Identifies the writer of the letter.

l. _____ Is used when the sender of the letter is representing the company.

m. _____ The date the letter was written.

n. _____ Includes three sections.

o. _____ Used to identify the sender and the typist of the letter.

p. _____ Used to notify the reader that a copy of the document is being forwarded to another party.

N. Company signature
O. Closing
P. Body of the letter
Q. Attention lines

4. All letter sections begin at the left margin, and proper spacing is applied between sections.
   a. Full-Blocked
   b. Blocked
   c. Semi-Blocked
   d. Square-Blocked
   e. Simplified or AMS

5. Date line is on the same line as the first line of the inside address and is right justified. Reference initials and enclosure reminders are typed on the same line as the signer's identification and are right justified.
   a. Full-Blocked
   b. Blocked
   c. Semi-Blocked
   b. Square-Blocked
   e. Simplified or AMS

6. Same as blocked with one change; paragraphs are indented five spaces.
   a. Full-Blocked
   b. Blocked
   c. Semi-Blocked
   d. Square-Blocked
   e. Simplified or AMS

7. Margins are the same as full-blocked, with the exception of dateline, complimentary close, company signature, and writer's identification.
   a. Full-Blocked
   b. Blocked
   c. Semi-Blocked
   d. Square-Blocked
   e. Simplified or AMS

8. Style is fast and efficient.
   a. Full-Blocked
   b. Blocked
   c. Semi-Blocked
   d. Square-Blocked
   e. Simplified or AMS

As the administrative dental assistant it is your responsibility to process outgoing mail. In the following scenarios, identify the type of mail service you would select.

9. You have just completed the quarterly newsletter (350 newsletters). The newsletters are bundled according to the specifications of the postal service.
   What type of postage has been used? _____

10. At the end of the day you have completed several insurance claims for the same carrier. It is important the claims arrive in the next 2 days.
    How will the package (under 2 pounds) be labeled? _____

    What is the current rate for this type of service? _____

11. Joel Curren has an appointment tomorrow at 4:30 pm with an oral surgeon. You have been asked by Dr. Edwards to send a referral letter and x-rays.
    What type of service will you use to ensure the information is received in time for his appointment?

    _____

12. Dr. Bradley has just seen an emergency patient of Dr. Coffee's and has prepared a report. The patient is due back in Dr. Coffee's office this afternoon for a follow-up appointment.
    What information do you need to send, and how will you ensure that it will arrive on time?

    _____

ACTIVITY EXERICSE

13. Complete the following tasks using the information below:
    - Write a referral letter. (Create letterhead using the examples in textbook Chapter 4 for Dr. Edwards.)
    - Use word processing software.
    - Select a letter style of your choice.
    - Use your initials in the reference initials.
    - Address an envelope. (Use a real envelope or draw a business envelope.)

Joel is being referred to Donald Payne, DDS, 23454 Tenth Street, Suite 234, Canyon View, California 91786, Attention Joan. The referral is for the extraction of teeth numbers 1, 16, 17, and 32. Joel is 18 years old and will be leaving for college in 3 weeks.

WHAT WOULD YOU DO?

You have been asked to create a guideline for the dental office on sending e-mail messages. In your guideline you need to cover the type of messages that should be sent via e-mail, examples of good subject lines, and how to get the response you want.

Hint: Do an Internet search on "how to write an effective e-mail."

Unscramble each of the clue words. Copy the letters in the numbered cells into the cells with the same number below the scrambled words. Solve the phrase at the bottom.

Business Letters

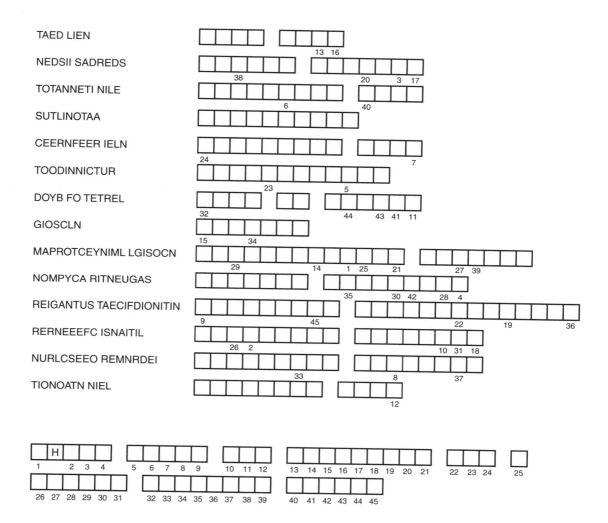

TAED LIEN

NEDSII SADREDS

TOTANNETI NILE

SUTLINOTAA

CEERNFEER IELN

TOODINNICTUR

DOYB FO TETREL

GIOSCLN

MAPROTCEYNIML LGISOCN

NOMPYCA RITNEUGAS

REIGANTUS TAECIFDIONITIN

RERNEEEFC ISNAITIL

NURLCSEEO REMNRDEI

TIONOATN NIEL

5 Patient Relations

INTRODUCTION

Patient relations include empathy, understanding, concern, and warmth for each patient. These concerns can be demonstrated in the way we communicate with the patient, the type of service that is provided, how members of the dental healthcare team relate to each other, and how problems are solved. Every aspect of the dental practice should be conducted with the understanding that the patient is "number one."

LEARNING OBJECTIVES

1. Compare and contrast the humanistic theory according to Maslow and Rogers. Relate the theory to patient relations.
2. List the stages that present a positive image for the dental practice.
3. Describe the different elements of a positive image and give examples.
4. Demonstrate different problem-solving techniques.
5. Examine different methods of providing outstanding customer service.
6. Discuss team strategies and personal strategies for providing exceptional patient care.

EXERCISES

1. Match the following statements with the corresponding stage:

   a. _____ Advertisement

   b. _____ Amount of information given

   c. _____ Answers to questions match individual needs

   d. _____ Appearance of the reception area

   e. _____ Attitude and professionalism meet expectations

   f. _____ Communication skills of the staff and dentist

   g. _____ Financial arrangements meet needs

   h. _____ How the telephone is answered

   i. _____ Name of dental practice

   j. _____ Office is easy to find

   k. _____ Talking with friends

   l. _____ Time spent waiting

   A. Investigation Stage
   B. Initial Contact Stage
   C. Confirmation of Initial Impression Stage
   D. Final Decision Stage

2. What can be done to ensure that patients' expectations are being met? List the eight points (summarize).

_____

_____

_____

_____

_____

_____

_____

_____

In the following scenario, the administrative dental assistant is faced with a typical daily problem. Michele Austin is a 32-year-old patient who has been scheduled three different times for completion of a root canal. Each time when you call and confirm the appointment, she finds some reason to postpone it. She has told you that her schedule at work is very busy and she cannot leave, that her daughter has a dance recital, and that she has to make final arrangements for the family dinner party. You have just called her for the fourth time, and this time, she informs you that she will be leaving on vacation next week and wants to wait until she gets back.

3. What steps would you take to identify the problem? (With information given in the scenario, use your imagination and list the problem or problems.)

_____

_____

_____

_____

_____

_____

4. Based on your selected problem, what steps will you take to solve this problem? Is there more than one way to solve the problem?

_____

_____

_____

_____

_____

5. Can the problem be prevented in the future? If so, how?

_____

_____

_____

_____

_____

6. Identify strategies that can be used by the dental healthcare team to provide outstanding customer (patient) service.

_____

_____

_____

_____

_____

_____

_____

_____

_____

7. Based on your personal experiences, which is the most important of these strategies (from Question No. 6), and why?

_____

_____

_____

_____

_____

_____

_____

_____

WHAT WOULD YOU DO?

You have been asked to work on a small team of colleagues (clinical assistant, dental hygienist, and associate dentist) to explore the development of a practice website. The practice is just opening a new location, and the primary purpose of the site is to introduce the dental practice to the community. You have been asked to give your opinion on the following:

1. What do you think should be included on the website?
2. What are the legal and ethical advertising guidelines the dental practice needs to follow?
3. Provide examples of websites that meet your criteria and explain why.

Hint: Do an Internet search for "dental websites" and search the American Dental Association (ADA) website for advertising information.

PUZZLE

Fit the letters in each column into the boxes directly above them to form words. Once a letter is used, cross it off. A black square indicates the end of a word. You will be able to find a completed quotation.

Dental Relations Quotation

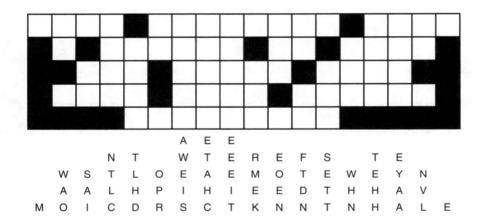

6 Dental Healthcare Team Communications

INTRODUCTION

A team can be described as a group of two or more members who work toward a common goal. Much as in a sports team, each member must understand and practice established rules and have a common goal. Developing an effective healthcare team requires a shared philosophy, excellent communication skills, the desire to grow and change, and the ability to be flexible while providing quality care for all patients.

LEARNING OBJECTIVES

1. Discuss the purpose of a dental practice procedural manual, and identify the different elements of the manual.
2. Categorize the different channels of organizational communication and identify the types of communication that are used in each channel.
3. Identify and discuss barriers to organizational communications.
4. Describe different types of organizational conflict and select the appropriate style for resolution.
5. Explain the purpose of staff meetings.

EXERCISES

1. List the main elements of a procedural manual.

2. Identify the four channels of organizational communication, and give two examples for each channel.

Identify the type of barrier to organizational communication that may result in the following scenarios:

3. Kim tells the office manager about a new idea she has that will improve the insurance billing process. The office manager decides not to tell the dentist about the idea. Classify the barrier. _____

4. Julie has a very full schedule as the receptionist. Kim, the insurance clerk, calls in sick, and tells Julie that the daily insurance claims must be processed by the end of the day and asks if she will take on the responsibility of completing the task. Classify the barrier. _____

5. Kim is told that she will not get paid for her sick day because she did not report the absence correctly. Kim questions the ruling because it is the first time she has been informed that there is a reporting policy. Classify the barrier. _____

6. Julie is excited about a new seminar that is being offered. She tries to explain the seminar to the dentist on his way out of the office to meet with the accountant. She is disappointed when he does not share in her excitement. Classify the barrier. _____

7. Organizational conflict can be described as _____ (conflict within the organization) and _____ (conflict between two or more organizations).

8. Define the four types of intraorganizational conflict.

   • Intrapersonal Conflict:

   _____

   _____

   _____

   • Interpersonal Conflict:

   _____

   _____

   _____

   • Intragroup Conflict:

   _____

   _____

   _____

- Intergroup Conflict:

_____

_____

_____

9. Identify and define the five conflict-handling styles, according to Rahim.

_____

_____

_____

_____

_____

_____

10. State the purpose of a staff meeting at the beginning of each day.

_____

_____

_____

_____

WHAT WOULD YOU DO?

Which style of conflict resolution would be appropriate for the following problems? (Support your answer.)

11. *Problem:* A new computer system is needed.

_____

_____

_____

_____

12. *Problem:* You don't like the color of the new uniform, and everyone else thinks it is great. (You will have to wear this color only once a week.)

_____

_____

_____

_____

13. *Problem:* Dr. Edwards takes 2 weeks off during the summer and closes her office. Her staff cannot agree on a vacation schedule for all of them; therefore, Dr. Edwards sets the date and does not offer any options.

_____

_____

_____

_____

14. *Problem:* Julie and Kim both want to leave early to get ready for the long weekend. One person will have to stay until 6 PM to check out the last patient. Julie agrees to stay only if Kim will open for her on Tuesday morning.

_____

_____

_____

_____

Search for the **BOLDFACE CAPITALIZED** terms seen in the list below in this word search puzzle.

Intergroup Communications

```
G N I T A N I M O D D A O L R E V O S T U L
N I N F O R M A L C H A N N E L L Y L V H W
I K T L E D B R A N K E R Q T Y E A E S E R
T G E O W Q N B N E L O L L V C N V N D Q G
A O R R Q W E F O T Y E W Q H O N O N F W P
R P G T D E S D I F N X A A I M A I A G A O
G K R N P R I L T N Y V Z T N P H D H H S I
E L O O O P O P A T U B A T T R C I C P D H
T A U C J I N H Z U F Z F R R O D N L O F V
N N P F Y J C D I J I U G J A M R G A I G L
I O Z O K D I G N N L Y Q N G I A T T U H A
K S Y N R U N H A Q T T Z B R S W R N Y J N
V R R A U J O G G A E R X V O I N W O T P O
U E W P H S R Z R S R E C B U N W E Z R O S
P P U S U O T X O R I D L V P G O Q I Q I R
U A T T A W C F R F N I A S G Q D W R W U E
O R A R L Q E T E C G S D F G T E E O E Y P
P T T K P R L Y T I M I N G W R R R H R T R
S N I J O D E U N W Q E R T Q D T T F T R E
I I U F K N L G I S D F G Y S S G F G G D T
K H X S W A E R T G H I O P D S R E T Y U N
F K L O P G D W E R T Y U I G F B C X Z F I
```

AVOIDING Style

COMPROMISING Style

DOMINATING Style

ELECTRONIC NOISE

FILTERING by Level

Formal **DOWNWARD CHANNEL**

HORIZONTAL CHANNEL

Inappropriate **SPAN OF CONTROL**

INFORMAL CHANNEL

INTEGRATING Style

INTERGROUP Conflict

INTERORGANIZATIONAL Conflict

INTERPERSONAL Conflict

INTRAGROUP Conflict

INTRAORGANIZATIONAL Conflict

INTRAPERSONAL Conflict

OBLIGING Style

RANK

STATUS

TIMING

UPWARD CHANNEL

Work **OVERLOAD**

7 Computerized Dental Practice Systems

INTRODUCTION

The use of computers in a dental practice is becoming standard. Computers help staff members to manage office functions, submit insurance claims, track patients, schedule appointments, and record treatments. It will be the duty of an administrative dental assistant to become familiar with and be capable of using a computer system.

LEARNING OBJECTIVES

1. Compare the three levels of function of dental practice management software and discuss their application.
2. List the functions to consider when selecting dental practice management software.
3. Discuss the role of the administrative dental assistant in the operation of a computerized dental practice.
4. Identify the different computer tasks performed by the administrative dental assistant.
5. Describe the importance of a computer system backup routine.

EXERCISES

1. Briefly describe the three levels of function of dental practice management software.

   Level One, Basic Systems: _____

   _____

   _____

   _____

   Level Two, Intermediate Systems: _____

   _____

   _____

   _____

   Level Three, Advanced Systems: _____

   _____

   _____

   _____

2. Identify the level of the dental practice management software at which the following functions can be performed. (*Note:* There may be more than one level.):

Function	Basic	Intermediate	Advanced
A. Word processing	_____	_____	_____
B. Electronic scheduling	_____	_____	_____
C. Retain demographic information	_____	_____	_____
D. Maintain clinical information	_____	_____	_____
E. Provide software security	_____	_____	_____
F. Process insurance information	_____	_____	_____
G. Personalize recall procedures	_____	_____	_____
H. Digital radiographs	_____	_____	_____

3. List the functions you should consider when selecting dental management practice software.

_____

_____

_____

_____

_____

_____

_____

_____

_____

4. Describe at least two reasons why dental practice management software is important to a dental practice.

_____

_____

Describe the functions of the management practice software package that are of use to each of the following members of the dental healthcare team:

5. Accountant: _____

6. Dental hygienist: _____

7. Administrative dental assistant: _____

8. Insurance clerk: _____

9. Describe the role of the administrative dental assistant in the operation of a computerized dental practice.

_____

_____

_____

_____

_____

_____

10. What are the advantages of using a computerized system?

_____

_____

_____

_____

_____

_____

11. List the daily procedures performed with the use of computerized dental software.

_____

_____

_____

_____

_____

_____

12. Describe the importance of backing up a computerized dental practice system.

_____

_____

_____

_____

_____

_____

13. Match the following computerized dental practice software terms to their definitions:

a. _____ Appears when additional information
   is needed

b. _____ Identifies software being used

c. _____ Provides information about current
   screen

d. _____ Arranges parts of screens in logical order

e. _____ Icons and buttons that identify
   commonly used features

f. _____ Identifies name of user

g. _____ Provides quick access to selected features

A. Menu Bar
B. Power Bar
C. Status Bar
D. Status Window
E. Main body
F. Title Bar
G. Toolbar

DENTRIX EXERCISE*

One of the key features of any practice management system is how patient files are managed. In Dentrix, this is done in the Family File. The Family File manages and stores both patient and family information, such as address, phone number, insurance coverage, and medical alerts.

In the Dentrix *User's Guide,* study the key elements of the Family File. (*Note:* The *User's Guide* is provided in electronic format on the Dentrix Learning Edition DVD and also saved on the Windows desktop when the Learning Edition is installed.)

a. Windows Areas in Family File
b. The Tool Bar
c. Family Member List

Selecting a Patient

Before you can perform many of the functions in Dentrix, you are required to select a patient.

1. In the Family File, click the **Select Patient/New Family** button. The Select Patient dialog box appears.

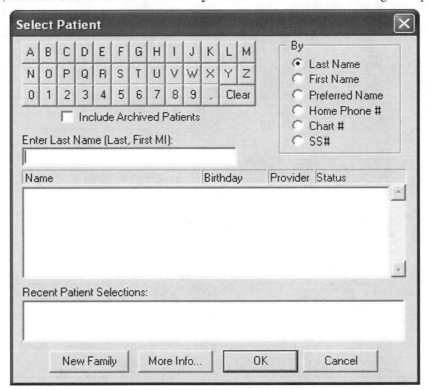

2. In the *by* box, select the criteria for the search.

3. Enter the first few letters/numbers of the selected search method in the field provided.

4. Select the desired patient from the list.

5. Click **OK.**

Search for the following patients:

1. Alice Gleason

    a. What is Alice's chart number?

2. Chart # KE0004

    a. Who is the patient?

3. Henry Myers

    a. List the other family members.

Editing a Patient's File

1. In the Family File, click the **Select Patient/New Family** button. The Select Patient dialog appears (see above).

2. In the *by* box, select the criteria for the search.

3. Enter the first few letters/numbers of the selected search method in the field provided.

4. Select the desired patient from the list.

5. Click **OK.**

6. To edit information, double click in the block that contains the information you need to change.

Edit the following information:

1. Karen Davis (head of household): New address (Double click on the address and bring up the Patient Information dialog box.)
    36487 N. Shoreline Drive
    Eastside, NV 11111
    Note: Once a head of household address is changed, you will see a pop-up box that asks whether you want to change all family members.

2. Lisa Farrer: New address and phone
    7649 Lincoln Court
    Southside, NV 33333
    879-3210 (home)
    768-6554 (work)

3. Michael Smith: New address
    231897 Northwestern Ave
    Centerville, NV 55555

Unscramble each of the word clue words. Take the letters that appear in the circle boxes and unscramble them for the final message.

Computerized Dental Practice

TILTE RBA

NEUM RAB

RIHDT RTAYP NVDREO

TOLO ABR

PORWE RAB

TUASTS RAB

DEBBAT SENCER

TUSTAS NOWWID

TSCAUNCO

8 Patient Clinical Records

INTRODUCTION

The function of the clinical record is to provide the dental healthcare team with information. It is the responsibility of the dental healthcare team to ensure that all aspects of the clinical record are accurate and easily accessible.

LEARNING OBJECTIVES

1. List the functions of clinical records.
2. List key elements of record keeping and describe the significance of each element.
3. Define the two types of accessibility of clinical records.
4. Discuss methods used in the collection of information needed to complete clinical records.
5. Identify the components of a clinical record and describe the function of each component.
6. Discuss the function of risk management.
7. Identify situations that lead to patient dissatisfaction.

EXERCISES

1. List the functions of clinical records.

_____

_____

_____

_____

_____

_____

_____

_____

2. List the three manners in which electronic clinical records are created and stored.

_____

_____

_____

3. List and describe the three HIPAA Security Standards that apply to electronic clinical records.

_____

_____

_____

4. List the key elements of record keeping and describe the significance of each element.

_____

_____

_____

5. Provide two definitions of the term *accessibility* as it relates to clinical records.

_____

_____

6. Identify the components of a clinical record.

a. _____ Components of the clinical record are organized and placed inside.

b. _____ Provides demographic and financial information.

c. _____ Documents probing, bleeding, mobility, and furcation conditions.

d. _____ Outlines the work that is going to be done, describes reasonable results, and alerts the patient to complications that may result.

e. _____ Estimated cost of dental treatment and payment schedule.

f. _____ Necessary to document the medical needs as well as the dental needs of the patient.

g. _____ Used to update and record conditions at the time of each recall visit.

h. _____ Records treatment.

i. _____ Prioritizes treatment that needs to be performed.

j. _____ Logs letters sent and received.

k. _____ Authorizes release of information about the patient.

l. _____ Illustrates the current dental condition of the patient at the time he or she is first seen in the dental practice.

m. _____ Information about the patient's previous dental treatment.

n. _____ Plan derived from information collected in the clinical record.

A. Individual Patient File Folder
B. Treatment Plan Form
C. Telephone Information Form
D. Signature on File Form
E. Registration Form
F. Recall Examination Form
G. Progress Notes Form
H. Problem/Priority List
I. Periodontal Screening Examination Form
J. Medical History Form
K. Financial Arrangements Form
L. Dental Radiographs
M. Dental History Form
N. Correspondence Log
O. Consent Forms
P. Clinical Examination Form
Q. Acknowledgement of Receipt of Privacy Practices Notice

7. Identify the components of the patient clinical record that are necessary forms.

_____

_____

_____

_____

_____

8. Risk management is a process that
   a. organizes clinical records
   b. is mandated by state regulations
   c. identifies conditions that may lead to alleged malpractice
   d. is unnecessary in an organized dental practice

9. Major reason legal actions are decided in favor of the patient:
   a. A patient is right
   b. The dentist is guilty
   c. Dental assistant is unavailable to provide interpretation of clinical entries
   d. Poor record keeping

10. Characteristics of clinical record entries include all of the following except
    a. Signature, date, and identification number of person making the entry
    b. Use of standard abbreviations
    c. Consistent line spacing
    d. Marking an error and writing over

11. Which is an example of an objective statement?
    a. Mrs. Oliver is in a strange mood today; she wants to be seen only by Dr. Edwards.
    b. Mrs. Oliver said, "I want to see only Dr. Edwards today."

ACTIVITY EXERCISE

Preparing Clinical Records

Your assignment is to prepare a clinical record for four patients (information to follow). In each of the following chapters, you will be given an exercise that pertains to your patient and his or her clinical chart.

Step One: Select a method by which to organize your patient's clinical record. The objective is to maintain a separate record for each patient. You will need one of the following:

- Four lateral file folders, four fasteners (you can also staple the records)
- Four horizontal file folders, four fasteners
- One three-ring notebook, four dividers

* It is very important that you complete only the exercise assigned in each chapter.

Step Two: Prepare clinical records for the following patients using the blank forms supplied in the appendix at the back of this workbook (p. 123). Use the information given to complete the selected forms. Not all of the forms required for a clinical record will be included in the exercises. Where information is missing, leave the space blank.

12. Prepare a clinical record for Jana Rogers.
    Complete the following forms:
    - Registration Form
    - Clinical Examination Form
    - Treatment Plan Form

13. Prepare a clinical record for Angelica Green. Complete the following forms:
    - Registration Form
    - Medical and Dental Form
    - Clinical Examination Form
    - Periodontal Screening Form
    - Treatment Plan

14. Prepare a clinical record for Holly Barry. Select the forms you will need.

15. Prepare a clinical record for Lynn Bacca. Select the forms you will need.

JANA J. ROGERS
Patient Information

Patient .... Jana J. Rogers
Date of birth 3-12-97
If child, parent name .... Donald Rogers
How do you wish to be addressed ....
Marital status .... Single
Home address .... 8176 Hillside
City .... Centerville
State/zip .... NV 55555
Business address ....
City ....
State/zip ....
Home phone 261-555-6217
Business phone ....
Patient/parent employer .... Valley Construction
Position .... Foreman
How long .... 12 yrs
Spouse/parent name .... Doris
Spouse employer .... Solutions Group
Position .... N/A
How long ....
Who is responsible for this account .... Donald Rogers
Driver's license number C3261
Method of payment .... Insurance
Purpose of call .... Toothache
Other members in this practice .... Donald, Doris, and Jason
Whom may we thank for this referral .... Parents
Notify in case of emergency .... Sadie Rogers
261-555-3001

Insurance Information 1st Coverage (Head of House)

Employee name... Donald Rogers
Employee date of birth 2/8/59
Employer .... Valley Construction
Name of insurance co .... Prudential
Address .... P.O. Box 15078
Albany, NY 12212-4094
Telephone 800-282-0555
Program or policy # 88442
Union local or group VC
Social Security # 012-34-5678
Fee Schedule .... None

Insurance Information 2nd coverage

Employee name .... Doris Rogers
Employee date of birth 12/2/62
Employer .... Solutions Group
Name of insurance co. .... Principal Financial Group
Address .... 10210 N 25th Ave,
Phoenix, AZ 85021-3910
Telephone 800-328-8722
Program or policy # 88446
Union local or group .... Solutions Group

Social Security # 632-24-7654
Fee Schedule .... None
Provider .... Dennis Smith Jr.
Privacy request .... None
First visit 4/12

JANA J. ROGERS
Medical and Dental History Information

Medical information .... Normal (not necessary to complete for this exercise)
Allergies .... Penicillin
.... (enter in Med. Alert box on all appropriate forms for this patient)
Dental Information .... Normal (not necessary to complete for this exercise)

JANA J. ROGERS
Clinical Examination Information
Missing Teeth & Existing Restorations

2	MOD amalgam
13	O amalgam
14	B amalgam
18	DO amalgam
19	Sealant
30	MOD amalgam
1-16-17-32	Extracted

Soft tissue examination OK
Oral hygiene fair
Calculus moderate
Gingival bleeding none
Perio exam no

Conditions/Treatment Indicated

3	DO amalgam
15	OB amalgam
18	B composite
30	Apical abscess/root canal
30	Core buildup (pre-fab)
30	PFM (high noble) crown

JANA J. ROGERS
Treatment Plan

Date	Category	Tooth#	Procedure	Fee
4/12	Diagnostic		Examination (periodic)	35.00
	Preventive		Prophy	60.00
	Diagnostic		4 bite-wing x-rays	40.00
	Diagnostic		1 PAs (each additional)	16.00
5/17	Restorative	3	DO amalgam	85.00
5/17	Restorative	15	OB amalgam	85.00
4/24	Endodontic	30	Root canal	420.00
5/10	Restorative	30	Post and core (pre-fab)	210.00
5/10	Restorative	30	PFM (high noble)	720.00
			Total Estimate	1671.00

All fees used in this exercise are for illustration only and do not represent actual fees charged for the procedures.

ANGELICA GREEN
Patient Information

Patient .... Angelica Green
Date of birth 7/20/82
If child, parent name ....
How do you wish to be addressed .... Angie
Marital status .... Married
Home address .... 724 E. Mark Ave
City .... Northside
State/zip .... NV 22222
Business address .... 3461 N. Cramer Ave
City .... Northside
State/zip .... NV 22222
Home phone .... (261) 555-3004
Business phone .... (261) 555-6134
Patient/parent employer .... James Tayor, DDS
Position .... RDA
How long .... 4 yrs
Spouse/parent name .... Anthony Green
Spouse employer .... Pacific States
Position .... Accountant
How long .... 8 yrs
Who is responsible for this account .... Anthony
Driver's license number 60314
Method of payment .... Insurance
Purpose of call .... Toothache
Other members in this practice .... None
Whom may we thank for this referral .... Dr. Taylor
Patient/parent SS # 736-82-9176
Spouse/parent SS # 286-34-2212
Notify in case of emergency .... Grace Miller, 555-9909

Insurance Information 1st Coverage (Head of House)

Employee name .... Anthony Green
Employee date of birth 9-13-82
Employer .... Pacific States
Name of Insurance Co. .... Dental Select
Address .... 5373 S Green St
.... Salt Lake City UT 84123-5432
Telephone 800-999-9789
Program or policy # 95740
Union local or group .... Pacific States
Social Security # 286-34-2212
Fee Schedule   None

Insurance Information 2nd Coverage

Employee name ....

Employee date of birth ....

Employer ....

Name of insurance co ....

Address ....

Telephone ....

Program or policy # ....

Union local or group ....

Social Security # ....

Provider .... Paula Pearson

Privacy request .... No phone calls

First visit 3/6

ANGELICA GREEN
Medical and Dental History Information

Medical information .... Normal with following exceptions

Allergies .... Sulfa drugs and codeine (enter in Med. Alert box on all appropriate forms for this patient)
Sensitive to latex
Bleeds easily when cut

Dental information .... Complete as much information as you can about the patient

Aware of problem .... Bleeding gums when I brush

Clench and grind teeth .... Yes

Gums bleed .... Yes

ANGELICA GREEN
Clinical Examination Information
Missing Teeth & Existing Restoration

1	....	Missing
2		O composite
3		B composite
14		DO composite
16		Missing
17		Missing
32		Missing

Chief Complaint: Bleeding Gums

Soft tissue examination: .... Normal

Oral hygiene: .... Good

Calculus: .... Heavy

Gingival bleeding: .... General

Perio exam: .... Yes

Conditions/Treatment Indicated

L/L .... Periodontal scaling and root planing

U/L .... Periodontal scaling and root planing

L/R .... Periodontal scaling and root planing

U/R .... Periodontal scaling and root planing

Periodontal Screening Examination

Tooth	Buccal	Lingual	Mobility	Furcation	Recession
2	676	455	1	2	1
3	876	767	1	2	1
4	444	444	0	0	0
14	876	765	1	2	1
15	453	543	1	2	1
18	547	665	1	1	0
19	767	878	1	1	0
30	455	445	1	1	0
31	667	778	1	1	0

ANGELICA GREEN
Treatment Plan

Date	Category	Tooth #	Procedure	Fee
3/6	Diagnostic		FMX ....…......................................	90.00
3/6	Diagnostic		Comprehensive exam ....…...............	45.00
4/12	Perio	L/L	Periodontal scaling & root planing…........	175.00
4/12	Perio	U/L	Periodontal scaling & root planing	175.00
4/24	Perio	L/R	Periodontal scaling & root planing ….......	175.00
4/24	Perio	U/R	Periodontal scaling & root planing..........	175.00
			Total Estimate	835.00

All fees used in this exercise are for illustration only and do not represent actual fees charged for the procedures.

HOLLY BARRY
Patient Information

Patient .... Holly Barry
Date of birth 3/6/32
If child, parent name .... NA
How do you wish to be addressed .... Mrs. Barry
Marital status .... Widowed
Home address .... 3264 S. Vine St
City .... Westside
State/zip .... NV 44444
Business address .... NA
City ....
State/zip ....
Home phone .... (261) 555-2331
Business phone .... NA
Patient/parent employer .... NA
Position .... NA
How long .... NA
Spouse/parent name .... NA
Spouse employer .... NA

Position .... NA
How long .... NA
Who is responsible for this account .... Self
Driver's license number 36788
Method of payment .... Credit Card
Purpose of call .... New Denture
Other members in this practice .... Son
....Donald Rogers
Whom may we thank for this referral .... Donald
Patient/parent SS # 111-32-4356
Spouse/parent SS # .... NA
Notify in case of emergency .... Donald Rogers

Insurance Information 1st Coverage (Head of House)

Employee name ....NA
Employee date of birth ....NA
Employer ....NA
Name of insurance co ....NA
Address ....NA
Telephone ....NA
Program or policy # ....NA
Union local or group ....NA
Social Security # ....NA

Insurance Information 2nd Coverage

Employee name .... NA
Employee date of birth .... NA
Employer .... NA
Name of insurance co .... NA
Address .... NA
Telephone .... NA
Program or policy # .... NA
Union local or group .... NA
Social Security # .... NA
Provider .... Dennis Smith
Privacy request .... none
First visit 2/4
Fee Schedule   None

HOLLY BARRY

Medical and Dental History Information

Medical information .... Normal (not necessary to complete for this exercise)
Allergies .... NONE (enter in Med. Alert box on all appropriate forms for this patient)
SPECIAL NOTE .... Patient cannot sit for long periods of time, must get out of the dental chair and stretch every 60 minutes
Dental information .... Normal (not necessary to complete for this exercise)

HOLLY BARRY
Clinical Examination Information
Missing Teeth & Existing Restorations

1-16	Missing
17-19	Missing
29	MODLB Amalgam
U	Complete denture: Placed 1990 relined 3 times loose fitting
L	Partial denture: Placed 1985, broken clasp

Chief complaint: Lower right molar broken
Upper denture very loose

Soft Tissue Examination	Normal
Oral Hygiene	Good
Calculus	Moderate
Gingival Bleeding	None
Perio Exam	Yes

Conditions/Treatment Indicated

U	Complete denture
29	PFM High noble
L	Partial denture, metal clasp, and framework

HOLLY BARRY
Treatment Plan

Date	Category	Tooth #	Procedure	Fee
2/4	Diagnostic		FMX	90.00
2/4	Diagnostic		Examination (limited)	35.00
4/12	Restorative	29	PFM	650.00
	Prostho		Complete maxillary denture	950.00
4/30	Prostho		Mandibular partial denture,	
		17-19	Cast metal framework	1050.00
			Total Estimate	2775.00

All fees used in this exercise are for illustration only and do not represent actual fees charged for the procedures.

LYNN BACCA
Patient Information

Patient	Lynn Bacca
Date of birth	8/12/2002
If child, parent name	Chuck Bacca
How do you wish to be addressed	Lynn
Marital status	Child
Home address	1812 Harman Dr.
City	Southside
State/zip	NV 33333
Business address	34655 VIP Parkway
City	Westside
State/zip	NV 44444
Home phone	(261) 555-3421
Business phone	(261) 555-6210

Patient/parent employer .... Diamond Welding
Position .... Production Manager
How long .... 8 yrs
Spouse/parent name .... Fern Bacca
Spouse employer .... Columbia Healthcare
Position .... Speech Pathologist
How long .... 5 yrs
Who is responsible for this account .... Father
Driver's license number 878765
Method of payment .... Insurance
Purpose of call .... Exam
Other members in this practice .... Parents, Brother Steve
Whom may we thank for this referral .... Aunt, Evelyn Evatt
                                                                                                                       3245 S. Spring St
                                                                                                                       Canyon View, CA 91711
Notify in case of emergency .... Parent

Insurance Information 1st Coverage (Head of House)

Employee name .... Chuck Bacca
Employee date of birth 7/27/77
Employer .... Diamond Welding
Name of insurance co .... Delta Dental Plan
Address .... PO Box 7736
                                                                                                                       San Francisco CA 94120
Telephone 415-972-8300
Program or policy # 12121
Union local or group .... Diamond
Social Security # 026-81-9217
Fee Schedule   None

Insurance Information 2nd Coverage

Employee name .... Fern Bacca
Employee date of birth 7/5/80
Employer .... Columbia Healthcare
Name of insurance co .... Connecticut General
Address .... PO Box 1650
                                                                                                                       Visalia, CA 93279
Telephone 800-252-2091
Program or policy # 55001
Union local or group .... Columbia
Social Security # 213-90-7148
Fee Schedule   None
Provider .... Brenda Childs
Privacy request .... None
First visit 4/12

LYNN BACCA

Medical and Dental History Information

Medical information .... Normal (not necessary to complete for this exercise)
Allergies .... (enter in Med. Alert box on all appropriate forms for
                                                                                     this patient)
Dental information .... Normal (not necessary to complete for this exercise)

LYNN BACCA

Clinical Examination Information

Missing Teeth and Existing Restorations

No Existing Restorations or Missing Teeth

Soft tissue examination: .... Normal
Oral hygiene: .... Good
Calculus: .... None
Gingival bleeding: .... None
Perio exam: .... No

Conditions/ Treatment Indicated

3 .... Sealant
14 .... Sealant
19 .... Sealant
30 .... Sealant

LYNN BACCA

Treatment Plan

Date #	Category	Tooth	Procedure	Fee
4/12	Diagnostic		BW X-Rays (4)	40.00
	Diagnostic		2 ANT PA's	14.00
	Preventive		Prophy and Fluoride TX	54.00
4/24	Preventive	3	Sealant	32.00
	Preventive	14	Sealant	32.00
	Preventive	19	Sealant	32.00
	Preventive	30	Sealant	32.00

Total Estimate 236.00

All fees used in this exercise are for illustration only and do not represent actual fees charged for the procedures.

Creating a New Family

To add a new family into the Learning Edition, you must create a file for the head-of-house. Once the head-of-house has been entered, you can add each additional family member to the family. *Note:* If the head-of-house is not a patient, change the status from *patient* to *nonpatient* (located in the drop down menu in the *Status* field). For detailed information on how to complete the head-of-house Information box, refer to the Dentrix *User's Guide,* Family File – Adding a New Family (Account). (*Note:* The *User's Guide* is provided in electronic format on the Dentrix Learning Edition DVD and also saved on the Windows desktop when the Learning Edition is installed.)

To create a file for the head-of house:

1. In the Family File, click the **Select Patient/New Family** button. The Select Patient dialog appears.

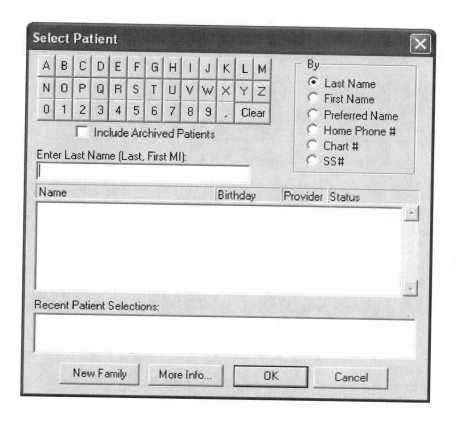

---

*Dentrix exercises based on content and screen captures courtesy Henry Schein Practice Solutions, American Fork, Utah.

2. Click **New Family**. The Head-of House Information dialog box appears.

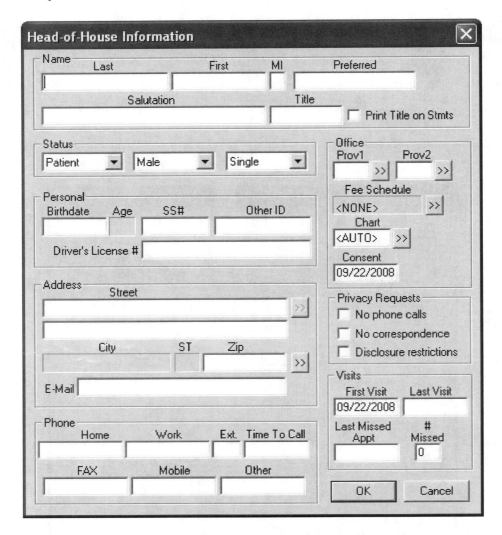

(*Note:* The Head-of-House and the Patient Information dialog boxes have the same fields, but the titles are different to inform you to enter the head-of-house's or new family member's information)

Adding Family Members

Follow these steps after you have entered all the information related to the head-of-house:

1. Click the **Add Family Member** button on the toolbar. The Patient Information dialog box appears. The last name, provider, home phone number, and address default to the information entered for the head-of-house file.

2. Enter Family Member information in the appropriate fields. *Note:* Refer to the Dentrix *User's Guide* Family File – Adding a New Family (Account) section for a complete explanation of each field.

Assigning Insurance

Note: To assign insurance to a patient, the insurance subscriber must be listed as a family member in the patient's Family File. If the subscriber is not a patient, set the status to *Nonpatient* in the subscriber's patient information.

Subscriber

1. From the Family File, select the patient/subscriber.

2. Double click the **Primary Dental Insurance** block. The Insurance Information dialog box appears.

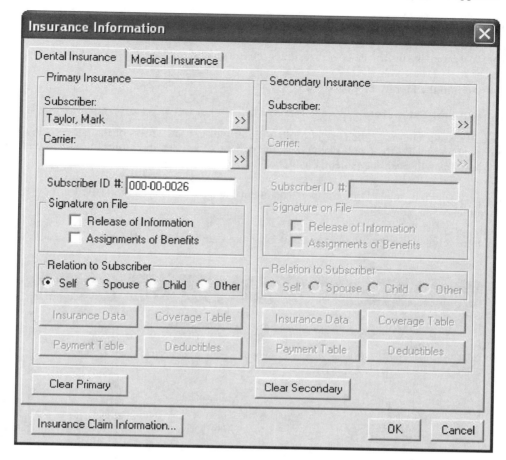

3. Click the **Search** button next to **Carrier**. The Select Primary Dental Insurance Plan dialog box appears.

4. Select a search option. Enter the first few letters or numbers of the selected option (carrier name, group plan, etc.).

5. Select the correct carrier and click OK to return to the Insurance Information dialog box. *Note:* If the carrier is not listed, click **New** and add the insurance carrier.

6. Select **Release of Information** and **Assignments of Benefits.**

7. Enter the subscriber's ID (sometimes the social security number) in the field provided.

8. Select Self, Spouse, Child, or Other as the patient's relation to the subscriber.

9. Click **OK** to return to the Family File.

Patient (Nonsubscriber)

1. From the Family File, select the patient.

2. Double click the **Primary Dental Insurance** block. The Insurance Information dialog box appears (see above).

3. Click the **Search** button next to **Subscriber**. The Select Primary Subscriber dialog box appears.

4. Select the primary subscriber and click **OK** to return to the Insurance Information dialog box. Note: If the subscriber is not listed, you will need to add him or her as a patient before you can continue.

5. Select **Release of Information** and **Assignments of Benefits.**

6. Select Self, Spouse, Child or Other as the patient's relation to the subscriber.

7. If the patient has secondary insurance coverage, enter the information in the *Secondary Insurance* box.

8. Click **OK** to return to the Family File.

Creating a Pretreatment Estimate

1. Click the **Select Patient** button on the Ledger toolbar. Enter the first few letters of the patient's last name. Select the desired patient and click **OK.** *Note:* If you have the patient's file open in Family File, select the Ledger button from the tool bar; this will open the patient's ledger.

2. From the Ledger menu bar, select Options, then Treatment Plan. *Note:* The Ledger Title Bar now reflects that you are in the Treatment Plan View.

3. To add procedures, click the **Enter Procedure** button on the Ledger toolbar. The Enter Procedure(s) dialog box appears.

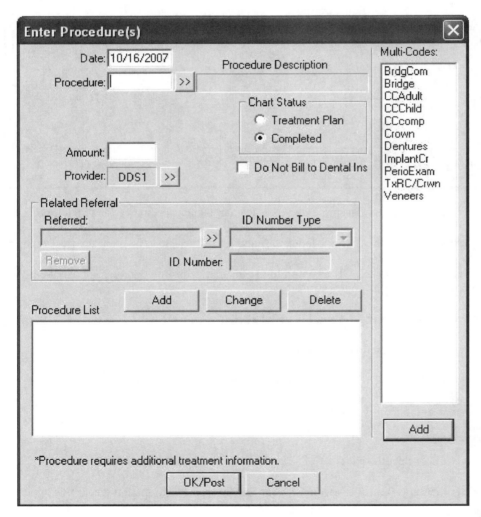

Add procedures to the Procedure List using individual codes or selecting the search button. Select the appropriate ADA Category. All procedure codes assigned to that category are displayed in the Procedure List. Select the desired code and click **OK.**

54

4. If the procedure code requires additional treatment information such as surface, tooth number, or quadrant, you should enter those now.

5. Once a procedure code has been selected a fee will be automatically assigned according to the fee schedule on file. However, you can enter a different fee in the **Amount** field.

6. Click **Add** to add this procedure to the Procedure Pane.

7. Repeat steps 1 through 6 for all procedures.

8. When all procedures have been listed click **OK/POST**.

Dentrix Patient Exercises

For this exercise, you will use the same information you used in Workbook Chapter 8, Activity Exercise to create clinical records for Jana Rogers, Angelica Green, Holly Barry, and Lynn Bacca.

1. Prepare a Family File for the Rogers family.

   A. Create a New Family with Donald Rogers as head-of-house (provider DDS2).
   Note: Assign subscriber insurance information by double clicking on the Insurance Information Block (see directions above).
   B. Add Doris as a new family member (see directions above to assign subscriber insurance information).
   C. Add Jana as a new family member (see directions above to assign insurance).
   D. Create a pretreatment estimate for Jana (see directions above).

2. Prepare a Family File for the Green family.

   A. Create a New Family with Anthony Green as H/H (*note:* Anthony is not a patient). Assign subscriber insurance information.
   B. Add Angelica as a new family member and assign insurance.
   C. Create a pretreatment estimate for Angelica.

3. Prepare a Family File for Holly Barry.

   A. Create a New Family with Holly as H/H and patient.
   B. Create a pretreatment estimate for Holly.

4. Prepare a Family File for the Bacca family.

   A. Create a New Family with Chuck as H/H. Assign subscriber insurance information.
   B. Add Fern as a new family member and assign subscriber insurance information.
   C. Add Lynn as a new family member (*note:* Do not do a pretreatment plan for Lynn).

5. Check the total estimate for each patient on the worksheet in the workbook. Do the figures match the total estimate on the patient's treatment plan? (*Hint:* If the totals do not match, did you change the fee when entering the procedure information?) Correct any figures that are not correct. Print out a copy of each patient's treatment plan. (See the Dentrix *User's Guide* for instructions on printing the treatment plan.)

Each letter of the alphabet has been assigned a number (e.g., O = 17). Working back and forth, solve the following quote from the chapter. *Hint:* Look for common words first (e.g., *a, an, the, of*).

Risk Management

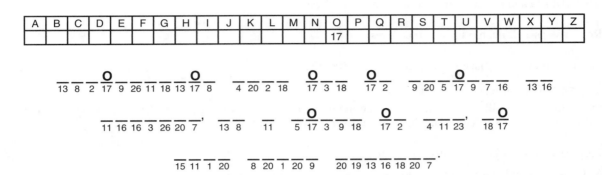

9 Information Management

INTRODUCTION

The responsibilities of the administrative dental assistant in the management of information do not end after the collection of data. These responsibilities continue, with proper storage and retrieval of information, files, and records. A systematic approach to filing is important to guarantee the integrity and safety of all documents.

LEARNING OBJECTIVES

1. List and describe the five filing methods outlined in this chapter.
2. Classify personal names according to ARMA (a not-for-profit professional organization and the authority on management of records and information) Simplified Filing Standard Rules by correctly indexing names as they will appear on filing labels.
3. List the types of filing methods used for filing accounts payable, accounts receivable, bank statements, and financial reports, as well as personnel records.
4. Describe methods that can be used for filing patient information.
5. Prepare a new patient's clinical record for filing.
6. Prepare a business document for filing.

EXERCISES

1. List the five basic filing methods.

_____

_____

_____

_____

_____

2. Define the following:

Indexing: _____

_____

_____

Filing unit: _____

_____

_____

Filing segment: _____

_____

_____

3. Using the personal name rule, identify which information will be placed in the following:

Unit 1 _____

Unit 2 _____

Unit 3 _____

Unit 4 _____

4. Using the business rule, identify which information will be placed in the following:

Unit 1 _____

Unit 2 _____

Unit 3 _____

Unit 4 _____

5. When a numeric filing system is used for patient records, a key component in locating the record is
   a. charts are arranged numerically
   b. charts are color-coded
   c. charts are randomly assigned numbers
   d. charts are cross-referenced

6. Geographic category records are filed according to
   a. Zip code
   b. area code
   c. city
   d. state
   e. all of the above

7. Subject filing is a method of filing strictly by subject. True or false, and why?

_____

_____

_____

8. Which method indexes by date?

_____

9. **Matching:** Identify the method of filing that would be used when a system is established for the following types of business documents. If a system uses two methods, list the primary location first, and the secondary method second. For example: Personnel files are first filed by subject (primary location) and then filed alphabetically by employee (secondary method). The answer will be S/A.

a. ___/___Accounts payable

b. ___/___Accounts receivable (ledger)

c. ___/___Bank statements

d. ___/___Financial reports

e. ___/___Personnel records

f. ___/___Payroll records

g. ___/___Tax records

h. ___/___Business reports

i. ___/___Insurance reports (business)

j. ___/___Insurance claims (patient)

k. ___/___Professional correspondence

l. ___/___Patient information

S. Subject
G. Geographic
A. Alphabetical
N. Numerical
C. Chronological

10. Maintaining an active filing system requires the removal of inactive records and documents. Identify two types of transfer methods and briefly describe how each method works.

_____

_____

_____

_____

_____

11. List the six basic rules for properly indexing names for filing.

_____

_____

_____

_____

_____

_____

12. For additional practice, complete Chapter 9, Critical Thinking Question 2.

_____

_____

_____

_____

ACTIVITY EXERCISE

Complete the preparation of clinical records for the following patients. Follow the guidelines listed in the text. (See Anatomy of an Indexed File Folder, p. 147)

13. Jana Rogers

14. Angelica Green

15. Holly Barry

16. Lynn Bacca

WHAT WOULD YOU DO?

You have been asked to write the new office policy for safeguarding patients clinical records (paper or electronic, your choice). You will need to research HIPAA policy and procedures. How will this be applied to a dental office?

1. Identify the type of records you will be addressing in your procedure guide (electronic or paper).
2. Research the HIPPA Policy for your selected choice.
3. Write a HIPAA Procedures Guide to be used in a dental office.

Using the clues below, fill in the crossword puzzle.

Filing Methods

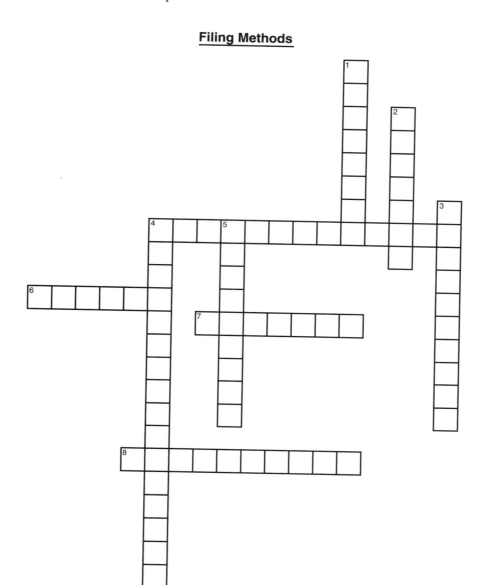

Across

4. Used to locate materials by date, month, or year
6. Used to divide filing systems into small sections
7. Filing method used for very large numbers of records
8. Categorizes records according to a location

Down

1. Arrangement of a name, subject, or number
2. Used to retrieve information according to topic
3. Follows strict rules standardized by the Association of Records Managers and Administrators
4. Identifies what other names (or name) a record is filed under
5. Used to fill the space occupied by a file that has been removed

10 Dental Patient Scheduling

INTRODUCTION

Developing and implementing an organized, functional schedule for a dental practice requires time, experience, and the cooperation of the entire dental healthcare team.

LEARNING OBJECTIVES

1. Describe the mechanics of scheduling.
2. Identify criteria required for matrixing an appointment book and electronic scheduler. Apply the criteria selected and properly matrix an appointment book and set up an electronic scheduler.
3. Discuss different methods used to identify when specific procedures should be scheduled.
4. List the criteria for making an appointment book entry (manual and electronic).
5. Discuss the seven different scenarios of appointment scheduling and formulate an action plan to solve the problems.
6. List the steps to be followed in making an appointment (manual and electronic).
7. Fill out an appointment card and a daily schedule.
8. Describe the use of a call list.
9. List the steps involved in performing the daily routine associated with the appointment schedule.

EXERCISES

1. If an appointment book has four time slots per hour, each time slot represents _____.
   a. 10 minutes
   b. 15 minutes
   c. 20 minutes
   d. 30 minutes

2. The dentist tells you that Judy will need 9 units for her next appointment (you are scheduling at 10-minute intervals). How long will Judy's appointment be?
   1. 1 hour
   b. 1 hour 10 minutes
   c. 1 hour 20 minutes
   d. 1 hour 30 minutes

3. A column in an appointment book is assigned to
   a. individual practitioner
   b. treatment room
   c. used for information
   d. all of the above

4. List the four steps involved in scheduling a follow-up appointment for a patient.

_____

_____

_____

_____

5. Place the following tasks in order. Place the number 1 in front of the first task to be completed, 2 before the second, and so on.

a. _____ Check patients' charts for any information that may not have been included on the schedule, such as need for premedication, payments due, or updated insurance and medical information.

b. _____ Confirm or remind patients of their upcoming appointments.

c. _____ Confirm the return of laboratory work.

d. _____ Give patients' clinical records to the dental assisting staff to review before they see the patients.

e. _____ Keep the dental healthcare team and patients informed of any changes that will affect their schedules.

f. _____ Pull the patients' clinical records, and review the procedures that are going to be completed the following day.

g. _____ Spend 5 to 10 minutes with the dental healthcare team to review the daily schedule.

h. _____ Type the daily schedule (or print out from the computer).

i. _____ Update schedules throughout the day as changes occur.

j. _____ Use the call list to fill any openings in the day's schedule.

6. List the criteria for making an appointment book entry. (See Anatomy of an Appointment Book Page, pp. 156-157).

_____

_____

_____

_____

_____

_____

ACTIVITY EXERCISE

You will need the clinical records you have completed for the following patients:

Jana Rogers
Angelica Green
Holly Barry
Lynn Bacca

7. Matrix an appointment book page (see pp. 156-157) for one day, April 12. There are four dentists and an expanded function dental assistant (EFDA) who have patients. How can you design the daily schedule so that each dentist does not have to share the treatment room with another provider while in the office? Use the following criteria:

a. Three columns: treatment room one, treatment room two, and treatment room three
b. 15-minute intervals
c. Include a 15-minute buffer period for emergencies for each dentist.

8. Schedule your patients. Check your patients' clinical records for detailed information on work to be completed on April 12 (treatment plan).

Jana Rogers	4 units with Dr. Dennis Smith Jr.
Angelica Green	8 units with Dr. Paula Pearson
Holly Barry	3 units with Dr. Dennis Smith
	2 units with EFDA for temporary crown
Lynn Bacca	2 units with Dr. Brenda Childs
	3 units with EFDA for coronal polish and fluoride treatment

(Review Anatomy of an Appointment Book Page, pp. 156-157 in textbook.)

9. Complete a Daily Schedule for April 12.

	Treatment Room 1	Treatment Room 2	Treatment Room 3
8 00			
15			
30			
45			
9 00			
15			
30			
45			
10 00			
15			
30			
45			
11 00			
15			
30			
45			
12 00			
15			
30			
45			
1 00			
15			
30			
45			
2 00			
15			
30			
45			
3 00			
15			
30			
45			
4 00			
15			
30			
45			
5 00			
15			
30			
45			
6 00			
15			
30			
45			

10. Complete an appointment card for each patient.

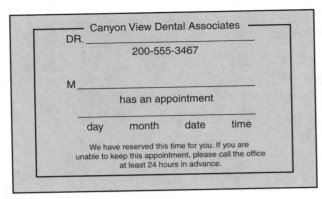

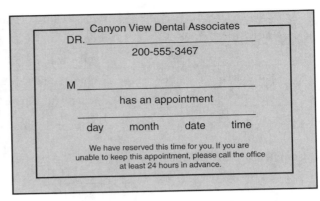

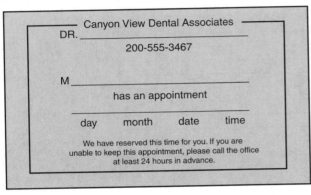

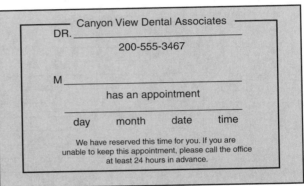

DENTRIX EXERCISE*

The Dentrix Appointment Book (or any electronic scheduler) is an essential component of the practice management software program. The electronic appointment book allows you to track appointments, color-code providers, procedures, and operatories, print route slips, and communicate vital patient information. In the following exercises you will

1. Set up your practice schedule

2. Schedule appointments for new and existing patients
   Before you begin the appointment book setup, you may find it helpful to review the Dentrix *User's Guide*, Appointment Book (specifically, Using Appointment Book). (*Note*: The *Dentrix User's Guide* is provided in electronic format on the Dentrix Learning Edition DVD and is saved on the Windows desktop when the Learning Edition is installed.)

*Dentrix exercises based on content and screen captures courtesy Henry Schein Practice Solutions, American Fork, Utah.

Setting Up the Appointment Book

The **Practice Appointment Setup** options in Appointment Book allow you to customize your practice hours, some appointment defaults, and the time block size used.

To set up practice hours:

1. In Appointment Book, from the **Setup** menu, click **Practice Appointment Setup.** The **Practice Appointment Setup** dialog box appears.

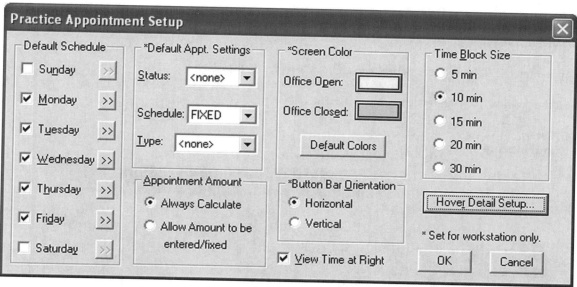

2. Dentrix allows you to schedule your appointments in 5-minute, 10-minute, 15-minute, 20-minute, or 30-minute intervals. Click the Time Block Size. (*Note:* In this exercise it will be a 15-minute interval.)

3. Dentrix defaults to a Monday through Friday work week.
   a. Select the days of the week the office is usually open. (*Note:* For this exercise the office is open Monday through Friday.)
   b. Clear the days the office is closed.

4. You can set working hours for each selected day.
   a. Click the **search** button (>>) to the right of the day.
   b. To change the time range for a time block, click the Start Time or End Time **Search** button (>>) of the time block you want to change.

   Note: For this exercise, set the following times:

Monday	8:00 am-12:00 pm and 1:00 pm-5:00 pm
Tuesday	8:00 am-12:00 pm and 1:30 pm to 5:30 pm
Wednesday	10:00 am-2:00 pm and 2:30 pm to 8:00 pm
Thursday	10:00 am-2:00 pm and 2:30 pm to 8:00 pm
Friday	10:00 am-1:00 pm and 1:15 pm to 3:00 pm

   c. When finished click **OK**.

5. Specify the default settings you want the Appointment Book to use for each new appointment when it is created
   a. Set the default **Status** field to ??????.
   b. Set the default **Schedule** field to **Fixed.**
   c. Set the default **Type** field to **General.**

6. Under **Appointment Amount** for this exercise, select **Always Calculate.**

7. (Optional) Set the colors you want Appointment Book to display.

8. Select **Button Bar Orientation, Horizontal** or **Vertical.**

9. Select **View Time at Right**.

10. Click **OK.**

Setting Up Providers

To set up the provider hours:

1. In Appointment Book, from the **Setup** menu, click **Provider Setup.**

2. Select the provider for whom you want to set a schedule.

3. Click **Setup**.
   The **Provider Setup** dialog box appears.

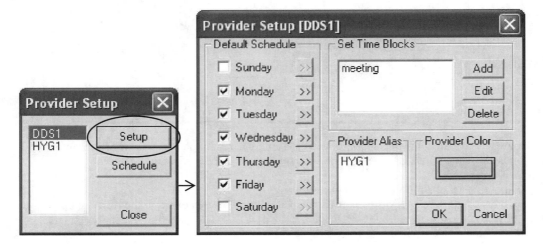

4. Select the days of the week the provider usually works.

5. Set the working hours for each selected day.
   Note: For this exercise each provider works the same hours as your office hours.

6. If desired, edit the provider's appointment book color in the Provider Color group box by clicking the color button.

7. Click **OK** to save changes.

8. Click **Close** to return to the Appointment Book

Scheduling Appointments

Scheduling appointments can be done in several different ways depending on the type and complexity of the appointment. More information is available on the following in detail in the Dentrix *User's Guide* in the Appointment Book section:

1. Scheduling (quick start)

2. Scheduling new patient appointments

68

3. Scheduling (comprehensive)

4. Scheduling continuing care appointments

5. Scheduling treatment plan visits

Scheduling (Quick Start)

The following instructions explain the simplest way to schedule an appointment.

1. Either by manually finding an appointment time or by using the Dentrix Find feature (discussed in the Dentrix *User's Guide*), locate and open schedule space.

2. In the Appointment Book, double click the appropriate operatory at the time you want to schedule the appointment. The **Select Patient** dialog box appears.

3. Enter the first few letters of the patient's last name.

4. Select the patient you want from the list, and then click **OK.** The **Appointment Information** dialog box appears. The **Provider** field defaults to the patient's primary provider.

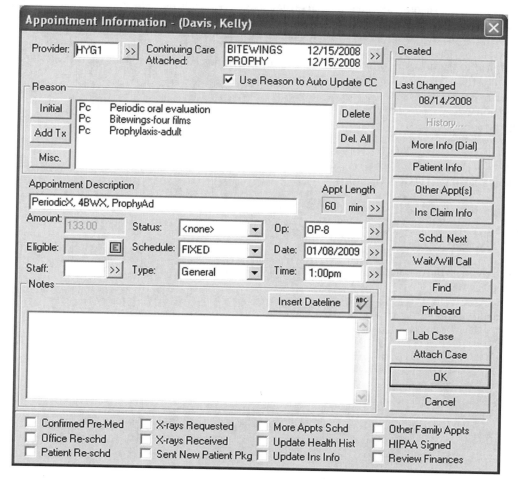

5. If necessary, click the **Provider** search button (>>) to select another provider for the appointment.

6. Under **Reason**, select a reason for the appointment using any of the following methods:
   a. If you are seeing the patient for work that would be done on an initial visit, such as an exam or a cleaning, click **Initial.** In the **Select Initial Reasons** dialog box, select the reasons for the appointment and then click **OK.**
   b. If you are seeing the patient for a treatment that was previously planned, click **Tx.** In the **Treatment Plan** dialog box, select the reasons for the appointment, and then click **Close**
   c. To add a new treatment-planned procedure, click **New Tx.** In the **Enter Procedure(s)** dialog box, click the **Procedure** search button (>>), select the procedures you want from the **Procedure Codes** dialog box, and then click **OK.** In the **Enter Procedure(s)** dialog box, click **OK/Post.** In the **Treatment Plan** dialog box, select the procedure you want for the appointment and click **Close.**
   d. If you are seeing the patient for a treatment that has not been planned, click **Misc.** In the **Procedure Codes** dialog box, select a **Category** from the list; under **Procedure Code List**, select the procedure code you want; and then click **OK.**

7. Once you have entered a reason, Dentrix automatically assigns a length of time to the appointment.
   a. To change the length, click the **Appt Length** search button>>.
   b. In the **Appointment Time Pattern** dialog box, click the right arrow to increase or the left arrow to decrease the number of minutes needed, and then click **OK.**

8. Click **OK** to save any changes you have made and close the **Appointment Information** dialog box.

Dentrix Patient Exercises

For this exercise you will schedule the appointments listed below. Schedule all the patients for the same day. *Note:* You have already set up treatment plans for Jana Rogers, Angelica Green, and Holly Barry. It is also important to assign the correct provider for the procedure. Decide ahead of time whether you will be assigning an operatory to specific providers. For example, does the hygienist work out of one predetermined operatory? Are there specific operatories assigned to the different providers? Set up your operatories according to the criteria you select.

1. Jana Rogers (1 hour)
   a. Examination
   b. Prophy
   c. 4-bite wing x-rays

2. Angelica Green (2 hours)
   a. Periodontal Scaling (L/L & U/L)

3. Mrs. Barry (2.5 hours)
   a. PFM (tooth #29)
   b. Final Impressions for maxillary denture

4. Lynn Bacca (*Note:* You will need to check Lynn's paper chart for fees.)
   a. 4-bite wing x-rays
   b. 2 anterior PAs
   c. Prophy and Fluoride Treatment

Rearrange the tiles to form a statement.

Scheduling

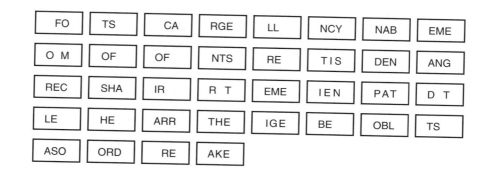

FO	TS	CA	RGE	LL	NCY	NAB	EME
O M	OF	OF	NTS	RE	TIS	DEN	ANG
REC	SHA	IR	R T	EME	IEN	PAT	D T
LE	HE	ARR	THE	IGE	BE	OBL	TS
ASO	ORD	RE	AKE				

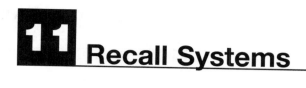

Recall Systems

INTRODUCTION

A recall system is an organized method of scheduling patients for examinations, prophylaxis, or other dental treatments. The success of a recall system depends on several factors: (1) Patients must be willing to return to the dental practice for follow-up care and examinations. (2) The dental practice must follow the procedure consistently to schedule patients at the prescribed time. (3) The dental practice must have an efficient method for tracking and contacting patients who fail to return at the scheduled time.

LEARNING OBJECTIVES

1. List the benefits to the patient of a recall appointment. List the benefits to the dental practice.
2. Discuss the elements that are necessary for an effective recall system.
3. List the different classifications of recalls.
4. Describe prescheduled, telephone, mail, and combination recall systems.
5. Describe the barriers to prescheduled, telephone, and mail recall systems.
6. Discuss solutions to the barriers of prescheduled, telephone, and mail recall systems.

EXERCISES

1. The success of a recall system is dependent on three factors. Identify these factors.

_____

_____

_____

2. List the benefits to the patient of a recall appointment.

_____

_____

_____

_____

_____

_____

_____

3. List the benefits to the dental practice of a recall system.

_____

_____

_____

_____

_____

_____

4. During a recall appointment, the dentist has the opportunity to reexamine the patient and evaluate his or her dental health. Other than a recall appointment for a prophylaxis, identify other treatment that may require a recall appointment.

_____

_____

_____

_____

_____

_____

5. Identify the following methods of recalling patients:

a. _____ This method is highly successful because patients have personally participated in the scheduling of their own appointment.

b. _____ Requires the mailing of recall cards to patients to remind them that they are due in the dental office for an appointment.

c. _____ Requires an assistant to call each patient before the month they are due for recall to schedule the appointment.

d. _____ Forms a partnership with the patient, and the recall appointment is worked around his or her preference.

A. Combination Recall System
B. Mail Recall System
C. Prescheduled Recall System
D. Telephone Recall System
E. Tracking System

WHAT WOULD YOU DO?

During a recent staff meeting, several issues have been raised about the effectiveness of the current recall system. The dental healthcare team has identified the following concerns:
- The hygiene schedule is booked 3 months in advance.
- There has been a decline in new patients.
- A review of the aging tabs on the clinical records reveals that a high percentage of patients have not been seen in the dental practice for one year or longer.

6. Your task as the administrative assistant is to evaluate these concerns by identifying the problem and presenting a possible solution. You will present your findings in the form of a report at your next staff meeting.

_____

_____

_____

_____

_____

_____

_____

_____

_____

_____

_____

_____

_____

DENTRIX EXERCISE (OPTIONAL)

Dentrix allows the use of multiple Continuing Care types (recall information). Review the information in the Dentrix _User's Guide_, Family File, section titled "Assigning Continuing Care." (_Note_: The Dentrix _User's Guide_ is provided in electronic format on the Dentrix Learning Edition DVD and is saved on the Windows desktop when the Learning Edition is installed.)

7. Assign a continuing care plan for Jana Rogers, Angelica Green, Holly Barry, and Lynn Bacca.

Search for the **BOLDFACE CAPITALIZED** words seen in the list below in this word search puzzle.

Recall Systems

```
T A Z K V L L R A E I F J K L N P
S N T V K I M B F S W Q T H J I O
V R E C A L L S Y S T E M I M R F
B Z I M U I O H R W Q A N A N T S
Z G C U T T D E U U I R R T V Y A
P R E Y O N I K R L Y E W Q T U Q
R Y T I P R I O P L J M F R E P W
E O W D J T X O J F A E R Y U L T
S P T R U D Z H P E H F J P H A F
C H E E F G C H T P D D M O Y U D
H K F T E O S C F R A S H I T T N
E L O H W L A Y N H T L D F S O N
D W I D Y Q D G E D T G L K T M B
U E K S R D B J R T G H K A G A P
L R O U T R F G H J L K P O C T H
E T R Y O P I T E L E P H O N E K
D R T I P K H F S Q W E R O K D R
```

AUTOMATED Recall System
MAIL Recall System
PRESCHEDULED Recall System

RECALL APPOINTMENT
RECALL SYSTEM
TELEPHONE Recall System

12 Inventory Management

INTRODUCTION

Ordering and managing supplies in a dental practice requires organization, communication, and the cooperation of the entire dental healthcare team. Inventory control is not limited to supplies in the clinical area. Those in the laboratory and business office must also be managed. Tempers flare and frustration levels climb when needed supplies are not readily available. To ease tensions between team members, a systematic and well-organized inventory management system must be implemented and practiced.

LEARNING OBJECTIVES

1. List the information needed to order supplies and products and discuss how this information will be used. Define *rate of use* and *lead time*.
2. Describe the role of an inventory manager.
3. Analyze the elements of a good inventory management system and describe how elements relate to the organization and overall effectiveness of a dental practice.
4. Compare the advantages and disadvantages of catalog ordering and supply-house services. Discuss when it is appropriate to use the two services.
5. List the information that should be considered before an order is placed for supplies and products.
6. Describe the different sections of a Material Safety Data Sheet and discuss what information is important to an inventory manager.

EXERCISES

1. List the information needed for ordering supplies.

_____

_____

_____

_____

_____

_____

_____

_____

2. List five responsibilities of an inventory manager.

_____

_____

_____

_____

_____

3. Define *rate of use*.

_____

_____

4. Define *lead time*.

_____

_____

5. Define *back order*.

_____

_____

6. A good inventory management system involves seven elements. List two elements and describe how they relate to the organization of an effective dental practice.

_____

_____

_____

_____

Using the scenarios below, determine whether to use a supply house or a catalog to order supplies. Identify which method you will use and explain why.

7. You have recently been hired as the new inventory manager for a large dental practice. After looking in the storage area, you realize that you do not recognize some of the products.

_____

_____

_____

_____

8. The dentist informs you that he has hired a new dental hygienist and wants to send out a mass mailing within the week publicizing her addition to the dental healthcare team. You will print the postcards in the office. When you check the inventory, you realize that you do not have enough postcards.

_____

_____

_____

_____

_____

Use the MSDS sheet for ProSpray Surface Disinfectant provided at the end of this chapter to answer the following questions.

9. What is the chemical name for ProSpray Surface Disinfectant?

_____

10. What physical state does the product have?
    a. gas
    b. liquid
    c. solid
    d. other

11. True/false: The product carries an odor. _____

12. If the product catches fire, how would you put it out?

_____

13. Is the product incompatible with another substance? If yes which one(s)?

_____

14. If the product comes in contact with your eyes, will it damage them? _____

_____

15. How would you protect your eyes when using this product?

_____

16. How should you dispose of the product?

_____

17. Where and by whom is this product manufactured?

_____

Search for the **BOLDFACE CAPITALIZED** words seen in the list below in this word search puzzle.

Inventory Management

```
E  G  N  I  S  A  H  C  R  U  P  L  W  U  H  E
Y  L  U  M  H  E  X  P  E  N  D  A  B  L  E  L
R  E  B  S  T  C  U  D  O  R  P  F  J  L  F  B
O  A  O  A  E  R  T  J  R  R  V  F  B  U  I  A
T  D  F  E  M  Q  E  A  D  I  M  A  M  Q  L  M
N  T  M  R  C  U  U  D  E  E  S  Z  S  W  F  U
E  I  N  A  A  P  S  I  R  O  D  N  E  V  L  S
V  M  R  E  T  U  R  N  P  O  L  I  C  Y  E  N
N  E  E  G  A  M  Z  S  O  M  K  D  H  N  H  O
I  M  X  A  L  S  I  H  I  C  E  C  X  O  S  C
O  E  B  R  O  D  A  N  N  K  N  N  A  B  E  D
A  G  T  O  G  S  P  I  T  Q  X  O  T  B  J  R
K  R  A  T  E  O  F  U  S  E  M  J  N  I  T  E
E  M  E  S  U  O  H  Y  L  P  P  U  S  U  J  D
S  E  I  L  P  P  U  S  K  S  N  G  D  U  Q  R
N  M  A  J  O  R  E  Q  U  I  P  M  E  N  T  O
```

BACK ORDER

CATALOG

CONSUMABLE

DISPOSABLE

EQUIPMENT

EXPENDABLE

HAZARDOUS Communication Program

INVENTORY

LEAD TIME

MAJOR EQUIPMENT

MSDS

NONCONSUMABLE

ORDER

OSHA

PURCHASING

RATE OF USE

REORDER POINTS

RETURN POLICY

SHELF LIFE

STORAGE Areas

SUPPLIES

SUPPLY HOUSE

VENDOR

Material Safety Data Sheet

Certol® International

ProSpray™
Surface Disinfectant

Product Number Prefix: PSC

6120 East 58th Avenue
Commerce City, CO 80022
Office (303) 799-9401
Fax (303) 799-9408
Toll-free (800) 843-3343
www.Certol.com
24-Hour Emergency Telephone
INFOTRAC: 1-800-535-5053
Importé au Canada par/Imported to Canada by:
Trans Canada Distribution Inc.
Mississauga, ON L5L 5Y7

ISSUE DATE: July 2010 (Supersedes: January 2008)

Certol International, LLC urges each recipient of the MSDS to read it carefully to understand the hazards associated with the product. The reader should consider consulting reference works or individuals who are experts in ventilation, toxicology and fire prevention, as needed to understand the use in the MSDS.

To promote safe handling, each recipient of the MSDS should: (1) notify anyone using the material of the MSDS information regarding hazards or safety; (2) furnish the MSDS information to customers purchasing the product; and (3) request the customers furnish MSDS information to all users.

Emergency and First Aid Procedures

Swallowing: Rinse mouth and throat thoroughly with water. Drink large amounts of water. DO NOT induce vomiting. Do not give anything by mouth to an unconscious or convulsing person. Seek medical attention immediately.

Skin Contact: Wash skin with flowing water or shower. If irritation persists, seek medical attention.

Inhalation: Remove the affected victim from exposure. Administer artificial respiration if breathing stopped. Seek medical attention immediately.

Eye Contact: Flush eyes with water for 15 minutes. If irritation persists, seek medical attention.

1. Identification

Product Name: ProSpray™ Surface Disinfectant
Chemical Name: Blend

2. Hazards

PRINCIPAL HAZARDOUS COMPONENTS	CAS #
O-Phenylphenol (OPP)	90-43-7
O-Benzyl-P-Chlorophenol (OBCP)	120-32-1

3. Physical Data

Appearance: Natural color
Odor: Lemon
Solubility In Water by Wt: 100%
Boiling Point: 212°F (100°C)
Freezing Point: Below 32°F (0°C)
Vapor Density: N/A
Evaporation Rate (BuAc = 1): <1
Specific Gravity (H₂0 = 1): 0.99 @ 68°F (20°C)
pH: 9.0 – 10.0 @ 68°F (20°C)

4. Fire and Explosion Hazard

Flash Point: Not flammable
Flammable Limits In Air: N/A
Special Fire Fighting Procedures: Wear self-contained breathing apparatus and protective equipment.
Unusual Fire And Explosion Hazards: None
Extinguishing Media: No special requirements

5. Health Hazard Data

COMPONENT	%	OSHA/PEL	ACGIH/TLV	LD₅₀ (Dermal Rat)	LD₅₀ (Oral Rat)
O-Phenylphenol	0.28%	N/A	N/A	> 5g/kg	2.7g/kg
O-Benzyl-P-Chlorophenol (OBCP)	0.03%	N/A	N/A	> 2.5g/kg	5g/kg

Effect of Overexposure:
Swallowing: Mild irritation of the mouth, throat and digestive tract
Skin Contact: May cause mild irritation
Inhalation: May cause mild irritation
Eye Contact: May cause irritation

6. Reactivity Data

Stability: Stable at normal conditions
Conditions To Avoid: Direct sunlight and cold below 45°F (7°C)
Incompatibility (Materials To Avoid): Acids, oxidizing and reducing materials
Hazardous Combustion or Decomposition Products: CO, CO₂ and other potentially hazardous fumes
Hazardous Polymerization: Will not occur

7. Spills or Leak Procedures

Steps To Be Taken If Material Is Released or Spilled: Absorb on clay, sawdust or other absorbent. Thoroughly rinse area with water. CAUTION: Spill area may be slippery. **Waste Disposal Method:** Dispose according to all local, state, and federal regulations.

8. Handling and Storage

Store closed container in a cool, dry, well-ventilated place away from incompatible materials. Do not store below 45°F (7°C). Keep out of reach of children.

9. Special Protection Information

Respiratory Protection: Not normally required. A mask or respirator may be used if vapor concentration is high.
Ventilation: Local exhaust or normal facility ventilation
Protective Gloves: Not required
Eye Protection: Safety goggles/face shield
Protective Clothing: Where contact may occur, wear protective clothing.
Other Protective Equipment: An eyewash station should be nearby and ready for use.

10. Regulation Information

Status On Substance List:
IARC: Does not list o-phenylphenol as a carcinogen.
NTP: Does not list o-phenylphenol as a carcinogen.
OSHA: Does not list o-phenylphenol as a carcinogen.
Chemicals listed as Carcinogen or Potential Carcinogen: National Toxicology Program; I.A.R.C. Monographs and OSHA do not list this product or its ingredients as carcinogens. o-phenolphynol produced urinary bladder tumors in male rats and liver tumors in male mice when fed exaggerated doses.
Federal EPA: 46851-5
Canada DIN: 02231483
State Right-to-Know:
SARA Section 311/312/313 OPP, OBCP

11. Transportation Data

Proper Shipping Name: None
D.O.T.: Unregulated Commodity

CHEMICAL WARNING LABELS
Required on containers, tubs, and bottles, which are filled from original containers with potentially hazardous substances.

Chemical Warning Label - Certol International, LLC
Product Name: ProSpray™ Surface Disinfectant
Hazardous Chemicals: O-phenyl/phenol, o-benzyl-p-chlorophenol
Personal Protection: Coggles and face shield
No wall reference is necessary.

ROUTE OF ENTRY	HEALTH HAZARD	FIRE HAZARD
✓ Inhalation	✓ Irritant	☐ Below 73°F (23°C)
✓ Ingestion	☐ Carcinogen	☐ Below 100°F (38°C)
✓ Eye absorption	☐ Toxic	☐ Above 100°F (38°C) & not > 200°F (93°C)
	☐ Sensitizer	☐ Above 200°F (93°C)
TARGET ORGAN	☐ Normal	✓ Will not burn
EFFECTS	☐ Material	**REACTIVITY**
✓ Respiratory		☐ May detonate
☐ Heart	**PHYSICAL HAZARD**	☐ Shock and heat may detonate
☐ Kidney	☐ Oxidizer	☐ Violent chemical change
✓ Eyes	☐ Acid	☐ Unstable if heated
☐ Skin	☐ Alkali	✓ Stable
☐ Prostate	☐ Corrosive	
☐ Blood	☐ Use no water	
☐ Liver	☐ Radioactive	
☐ CNS		
☐ Other		

Hazard rating corresponding to the NFPA Rating System.

4 - Extreme
3 - High
2 - Moderate
1 - Slight
0 - Insignificant

NFPA HAZARD RATING

HEALTH: 1
FLAMMABILITY: 0
REACTIVITY: 0

The information contained herein is furnished without warranty or legal responsibility of any kind. Employers should use this information only as a supplement to other information gathered by them and must make independent determination of suitability and completeness of information from all sources to assure proper use of these materials and the safety and health of employees.

PSC/MSDS/03 07/10

13 Office Equipment

INTRODUCTION

Office equipment helps the administrative dental assistant organize and perform tasks and save time by integrating different types of procedures. Equipment is selected on the basis of the needs of the staff. Equipment can be divided into two broad categories: equipment used to gather, transfer, and store information; and equipment used to create a working environment that is safe, organized, and functional.

LEARNING OBJECTIVES

1. List the components of a dental practice information system and explain the function of each component.
2. Categorize the different functions of a dental practice telecommunication system.
3. Describe the features of a telephone system, and explain how they can be used in a modern dental practice.
4. Design an ergonomic workstation. Identify important elements and state their purpose.

EXERCISES

1. List and define the components of a dental practice information system.

_____

_____

_____

_____

_____

2. List and briefly describe the features of a telephone system.

_____

_____

_____

_____

_____

_____

_____

_____

_____

3. List the functions of a telecommunication system and describe how it can be used in a dental practice.

_____

_____

_____

_____

4. List seven factors to consider when setting up an ergonomic workstation.

_____

_____

_____

_____

_____

_____

_____

5. Match the following terms to their definitions:

a. _____ Peripheral device used to activate commands

b. _____ Similar to a television screen

c. _____ Information needed for the computer to be able to function

d. _____ Used to back up information

e. _____ Main operating component of hardware

f. _____ Digitizes information from a document

g. _____ Produces a hard copy of information

h. _____ Most common input device

i. _____ Transfers information

A. CPU
B. Keyboard
C. Mouse
D. Scanner
E. Modem
F. Monitor
G. Printer
H. Storage device
I. Operating system

6. Define *intraoffice communications*.

_____

7. List the different types of intraoffice communication systems.

_____

_____

_____

_____

_____

_____

_____

8. List the types of office machines found in a dental practice.

_____

_____

_____

_____

_____

Define the following terms:

9. Ergonomics _____

10. Background noise _____

11. Lighting _____

WHAT WOULD YOU DO?

Ergonomic Problem Solving

12. Sally, the administrative dental assistant, is complaining of lower back pain. What should she check on her chair to rectify this problem?

_____

_____

_____

_____

13. Kevin, the business manager, is complaining of eyestrain. What can he do with his video display terminal to help alleviate the strain?

_____

_____

_____

14. Hope, the insurance biller, has been given a diagnosis of carpal tunnel syndrome. What can she do with her keyboard and mouse to help reduce the strain?

_____

_____

_____

PUZZLE

Unscramble each of the clue words. Copy the letters in the numbered cells to other cells with the same number to spell out a phrase.

Ergonomics

Clue	
NLPOIPAATIC WAFOTRES	
CRNOGKDBAU INSOE	
TAAD	
GOOCMNISER	
WAHADRER	
INTUP DIVCESE	
DKEDBAROY	
GIGNITLH	
DOEMM	
MESUO	
TUOPUT DESCIVE	
CANRNES	
REAWOFTS	
LAICUMTECONMONTEI	

1 2 3 4 5 6   7 Q 8 9 10 11 12 13 14   15 16 17 18 19

14 Financial Arrangements and Collection Procedures

INTRODUCTION

The responsibility for collecting fees is shared by all members of the dental healthcare team. The team will establish the policies and then follow them. The administrative dental assistant has the most visible task. After a treatment plan is drawn up, the administrative dental assistant will write the financial plan, present the plan to the patient, and then monitor compliance with the plan. If the plan is not followed, it is usually the administrative dental assistant who initiates collection procedures.

LEARNING OBJECTIVES

1. List the elements of a financial policy and discuss the qualifying factors for each of the elements.
2. Describe the different types of financial plans and explain how they can be applied in a dental practice.
3. State the purpose of managing accounts receivable. Describe the role of the administrative dental assistant in managing accounts receivable.
4. Classify the different levels of the collection process.
5. Place a telephone collection call.
6. Process a collection letter.
7. Interpret aging reports and implement proper collection procedures.

EXERCISES

1. Match the payment plan to its definition.

   a. _____ Payment is spread out over time

   b. _____ Payment is paid by third party carrier

   c. _____ Payment installments are paid directly to the dental practice

   d. _____ Payment is divided by length of treatment

   e. _____ Another form of payment in full. Payment amount will be discounted and deposited directly into the practice's account

   f. _____ Payment is made immediately after dental visit by patient

   g. _____ Payment installments directed by a loan company

   A. Insurance billing
   B. Payment in full
   C. Outside payment plan
   D. In-house payment plan
   E. Extended payment plan
   F. Divided payment plan
   G. Credit card
   H. Creative payment plan

2. List the six steps to be followed in placing a telephone collection call.

_____

_____

_____

_____

_____

_____

3. At what level in the collection process should a letter be written?
   a. Level one
   b. Level two
   c. Level three
   d. Level four
   e. Level five

4. List at least two requirements of a properly written collection letter.

_____

_____

5. Match the following time intervals with the level of the collection process.

   a. _____ 0-30 days   A. Telephone reminder

   b. _____ 30-60 days   B. Ultimatum

   c. _____ 60-90 days   C. Mailed reminder

   d. _____ 90-120 days   D. Statement

   e. _____ Longer than 120 days E. Collection letter

   f. _____ No response to letter F. Turning of account over to collection

                                      G. Friendly reminder

ACTIVITY EXERCISES

Use information located on the Treatment Plan for each of the following patients to complete a Financial Arrangement Form (located at the back of the workbook).

Jana Rogers

Holly Barry

Angelica Green

Lynn Bacca

Jana Rogers

Jana's parents both have dental insurance. After their combined benefits are calculated, it has been determined that the total benefits paid will be $1200.00.
   As the administrative dental assistant, you propose the following financial arrangements.
   Initial payment ....$ 75.00
   Insurance estimated payment $1200.00
   The balance is to be paid in three monthly payments.
   Use the completed Financial Arrangement forms to answer the following questions.

88

6. What is the total estimate of treatment? $ _____

7. What is the balance of the estimate due? $ _____

8. What is the monthly payment? $ _____

Angelica Green

Angelica is covered by her husband's plan. His plan will pay 60% of the total estimate of treatment. In addition, Dr. Edwards will give Angelica a 10% professional courtesy discount on the balance after the insurance estimate. It is agreed that Angelica will pay the balance in six monthly payments.

Complete a Financial Arrangement Form for Angelica, and use the information to answer the following questions:

9. What is the total estimate of treatment? $ _____

10. What is the insurance estimate? $ _____

11. What is the amount of the discount? $ _____

12. What is the balance of the estimate due? $ _____

13. What is the monthly payment? $ _____

Holly Barry

Mrs. Barry is a senior citizen and will receive a 12% senior citizen discount. She has made arrangements to pay the balance in full (credit card) on April 12.

Complete a Financial Arrangement form for Mrs. Barry and use the information to answer the following questions.

14. What is the total estimate of treatment? $ _____

15. What is the amount of the discount? $ _____

16. What is the balance of the estimate due? $ _____

Lynn Bacca

Lynn's parents both have dental insurance. The combined payment will be 100% of the total estimate for treatment, less a $50.00 deductible.

Complete a Financial Arrangement Form for Lynn and use the information to answer the following questions:

17. What is the total estimate of treatment? $ _____

18. What is the insurance estimate? $ _____

DENTRIX EXERCISE*

Dentrix provides you the flexibility to set up two types of financial arrangements: (1) Payment Agreements and (2) Future Due Payment Plans. Payment Agreements can be used when treatment has been completed, and the balance will be paid over time. Future Due Payment Plans can be used when treatment will be completed over time and you want to charge an account monthly.

For this exercise use the information in the Activity Exercises to complete a Payment Agreement for a patient.
 1. In the Ledger, select a member of the family for whom you want to create a payment agreement.

_____

*Dentrix exercises based on content and screen captures courtesy Henry Schein Practice Solutions, American Fork, Utah.

Chapter **14** **Financial Arrangements and Collection Procedures**

2. Click the **Billing/Payment Agreement** button. The Billing/Payment Agreement Information dialog appears:

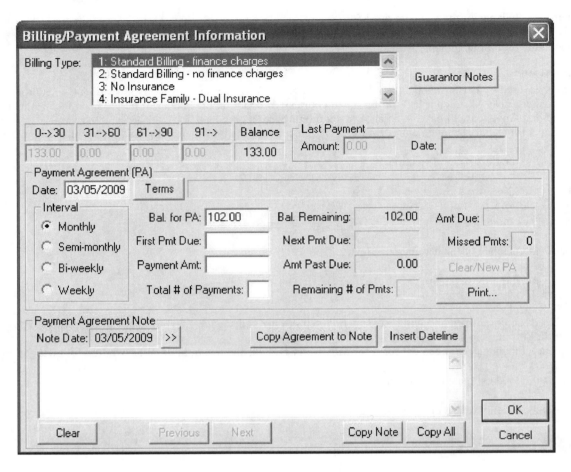

3. In the *Payment Agreement (PA)* group box, enter the agreement date in the **Date** field.

4. Click **Terms** to set up the terms of the payment agreement. The Payment Agreement Terms dialog appears:

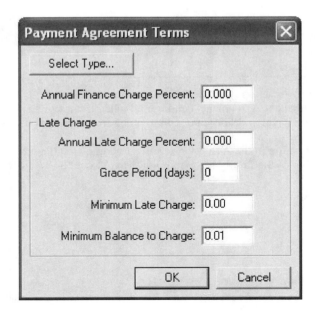

From here, terms can be set up either automatically or manually. For further instruction on how to complete this task, refer to the Dentrix *User's Guide,* Ledger, "Setting Up Financial Arrangements." (*Note:* The Dentrix *User's Guide* is provided in electronic format on the Dentrix Learning Edition DVD and also saved on the Windows desktop when the Learning Edition is installed.)

Patient Exercises

Complete a Payment Agreement for a patient (either Jana Rogers, Holly Barry, or Angelica Green).
    A. Print a Truth in Lending Disclosure Statement.
    B. Print a Coupon Book for Scheduled Payments (plain paper).

PUZZLE

Each letter of the alphabet has been assigned a number (e.g., E = 1). Working back and forth, solve the following quote from the chapter. HINT: Look for common words (e.g., a, an, the, of).

Financial Arrangements

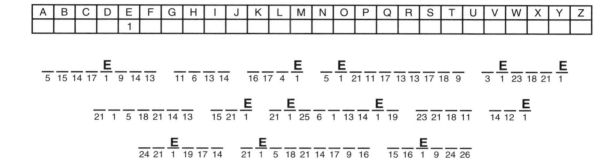

15 Dental Insurance Processing

INTRODUCTION

Before successfully processing an insurance claim form, the assistant will need to understand the types of available dental insurance coverage, insurance terminology, and ways to correctly code dental procedures. In addition, a clear-cut policy must be in place that outlines the requirements of the dental practice in relation to insurance billing and the patient's responsibilities.

LEARNING OBJECTIVES

1. Classify and identify the various types of insurance coverage.
2. Discuss the purpose of insurance coding and differentiate between categories.
3. List the types of insurance information required to determine insurance coverage.
4. Identify the different methods of filing insurance claims and discuss the responsibility of the administrative dental assistant in filing dental claims.
5. Discuss part 5B of the ADA Code of Ethics and identify how it applies to an administrative dental assistant.
6. Complete a dental claim form for manual submission.

EXERCISES

1. Match each of the following descriptions of types of dental coverage with the correct term:

a. _____ The benefits of this type of dental practice are a common name and the means for a large advertising budget.

b. _____ Programs that dictate to patients where they can receive their dental treatment.

c. _____ Programs in which the dental practice is paid a set amount for each patient who is enrolled in the program.

d. _____ List of procedures covered by an insurance company and their respective dollar amounts. These fees are the same for all dentists, regardless of location.

e. _____ Fee schedules that are calculated with distinct demographic information and criteria.

f. _____ Designed to contain the cost of dental procedures and services by restricting the types and frequencies of procedures and services and controlling fee schedules.

g. _____ Contract states that the dentist will use only the fee schedule preapproved by the third party. In exchange, the third party places the dentist's name on a preferred list.

h. _____ An organization that has been legally established by a group of dentists to enter into third party contracts.

i. _____ Accepts responsibility for payment of dental procedures and services for members. Will not cover services if the work is done outside of the organization.

j. _____ A method of payment that compensates the dentist according to individual services and procedures. Reimbursement is determined by established fee schedules.

k. _____ A method of payment that bypasses an insurance company and pays directly from a fund established by an employer.

A. Direct Reimbursement
B. Health Maintenance Organization
C. Individual Practice Association
D. Managed Care
E. Preferred Provider Organization
F. Table of Allowances
G. Capitation Programs
H. Closed Panel Programs
I. Franchise Dentistry
J. Fee for Service
K. UCR Plans
L. Union Trust Funds

2. Dental procedure codes are
   a. the same as medical procedure codes
   b. set by each insurance company to correspond with its coverage
   c. also known as SNODENT codes
   d. standardized by the ADA and accepted by all third party carriers

3. Maximum coverage can be described as
   a. the total dollar amount that will be paid for each service or procedure according to the stipulations of the insurance policy
   b. the total dollar amounts that an insurance company will pay during a year
   c. the total dollar amounts that an insurance company will pay for a family
   d. the total dollar amounts that an insurance company will pay for a lifetime

4. The percentage of payment will vary depending on
   a. the type of procedure
   b. the insurance contract
   c. where the patient seeks dental treatment
   d. all of the above

What Would You Do?

The administrative dental assistant may be faced with many ethical and legal issues regarding the billing of insurance. In the following scenarios, use the correct reference code taken from The American Dental Association's *Principles of Ethics and Code of Professional Conduct*, Section 5B, Advisory Opinions.

5. A patient has just discovered that he will no longer be covered for insurance benefits after the end of the month. The patient is scheduled for the second week of the next month to complete his treatment plan. When you check the schedule, you discover that the dentist is taking a week off and the schedule is already overbooked. The patient asks if you can change the date to the current month so the insurance company will pay.
   a. What are your options?

   _____

   _____

   _____

   _____

   b. If you change the date, what portion of the advisory opinion addresses this issue?

   _____

6. The last staff meeting focused on ways to attract new patients to the dental practice. Several ideas were discussed. One of the ideas suggested that patients who have dental insurance would not be responsible for their copayment after the insurance company paid. Your assignment is to research the idea and report back to the group at the next meeting. What will you report back at the next meeting?

   _____

   _____

   _____

   _____

ACTIVITY EXERCISES

For the following exercise, you will need your clinical charts for Jana Rogers, Angelica Green, Holly Barry, and Lynn Bacca. During the exercise you will be asked to complete an insurance claim form. For this exercise use the following chart of billing codes and provider information.

Dental Insurance Coding

Procedure	Dentrix Codes*
Periodic oral evaluation	X1407
Comprehensive oral evaluation	X1437
Periapical first film	X1507
Periapical each additional film	X1510
Bitewings – four	X1567
Prophylaxis-adult	X2397
Prophylaxis-child	X2490
Topical application of fluoride – child	X2495
Sealant – per tooth	X2638
Amalgam – 2-surface	X3047
Crown--porcelain fused to high noble metal	X4037
Endodontic therapy, molar	X4617
Prefabricated post and core	X5237
Periodontal scaling and root planing	X5628

*Note: The Dentrix Codes are placeholder codes designed to mimic the style of coding used by the American Dental Association (ADA). The actual ADA codes are copyrighted in the publication *Code on Dental Procedures and Nomenclature (CDT)* and appear only with the professional version of Dentrix.

Billing Dentist Information

Use the following information to complete all claim forms (all numbers are fictitious):

Mary A. Edwards, D.D.S.
4546 North Avery Way
Canyon View, CA 91783
987-555-3210
Provider ID#34567
TIN: 95-1234568
License#10111213

7. Who is responsible for primary insurance coverage for Jana Rogers? _____

8. Who is responsible for secondary insurance coverage for Jana? _____

9. Submit a completed primary insurance claim form (claim forms are located on the following pages) for Jana. Include treatment dated April 12, April 24, May 10, and May 17.

10. Who is responsible for primary insurance coverage for Angelica Green? _____

11. Identify the documentation that will be sent with Angelica's claim form. _____

_____

12. Complete a claim form for Angelica for the following dates: March 6 through April 24.

13. Who is the responsible party for Holly Barry? _____

14. What type of insurance coverage does Holly have? _____

15. Under the birthday rule, who is responsible for primary coverage for Lynn Bacca? _____

_____

16. When is the secondary insurance submitted for payment? _____

_____

17. Complete a primary insurance claim form for Lynn for April 12 and April 24.

18. Correctly document each clinical record.

ADA Dental Claim Form

HEADER INFORMATION

1. Type of Transaction (Mark all applicable boxes)

☐ Statement of Actual Services ☐ Request for Predetermination/Preauthorization

☐ EPSDT/Title XIX

2. Predetermination/Preauthorization Number

INSURANCE COMPANY/DENTAL BENEFIT PLAN INFORMATION

3. Company/Plan Name, Address, City, State, Zip Code

OTHER COVERAGE

4. Other Dental or Medical Coverage? ☐ No (Skip 5-11) ☐ Yes (Complete 5-11)

5. Name of Policyholder/Subscriber in #4 (Last, First, Middle Initial, Suffix)

6. Date of Birth (MM/DD/CCYY)	7. Gender ☐ M ☐ F	8. Policyholder/Subscriber ID (SSN or ID#)

9. Plan/Group Number	10. Patient's Relationship to Person Named in #5 ☐ Self ☐ Spouse ☐ Dependent ☐ Other

11. Other Insurance Company/Dental Benefit Plan Name, Address, City, State, Zip Code

POLICYHOLDER/SUBSCRIBER INFORMATION (For Insurance Company Named in #3)

12. Policyholder/Subscriber Name (Last, First, Middle Initial, Suffix), Address, City, State, Zip Code

13. Date of Birth (MM/DD/CCYY)	14. Gender ☐ M ☐ F	15. Policyholder/Subscriber ID (SSN or ID#)

16. Plan/Group Number	17. Employer Name

PATIENT INFORMATION

18. Relationship to Policyholder/Subscriber in #12 Above ☐ Self ☐ Spouse ☐ Dependent Child ☐ Other	19. Student Status ☐ FTS ☐ PTS

20. Name (Last, First, Middle Initial, Suffix), Address, City, State, Zip Code

21. Date of Birth (MM/DD/CCYY)	Gender ☐ M ☐ F	23. Patient ID/Account # (Assigned by Dentist)

RECORD OF SERVICES PROVIDED

	24. Procedure Date (MM/DD/CCYY)	25. Area of Oral Cavity	26. Tooth System	27. Tooth Number(s) or Letter(s)	28. Tooth Surface	29. Procedure Code	30. Description	31. Fee
1								
2								
3								
4								
5								
6								
7								
8								
9								
10								

MISSING TEETH INFORMATION

34. (Place an 'X' on each missing tooth)

Permanent: 1 2 3 4 5 6 7 8 9 10 11 12 13 14 15 16 / 32 31 30 29 28 27 26 25 24 23 22 21 20 19 18 17

Primary: A B C D E F G H I J / T S R Q P O N M L K

32. Other Fee(s)	
33. Total Fee	

35. Remarks

AUTHORIZATIONS

36. I have been informed of the treatment plan and associated fees. I agree to be responsible for all charges for dental services and materials not paid by my dental benefit plan, unless prohibited by law, or the treating dentist or dental practice has a contractual agreement with my plan prohibiting all or a portion of such charges. To the extent permitted by law, I consent to your use and disclosure of my protected health information to carry out payment activities in connection with this claim.

X_____
Patient/Guardian signature   Date

37. I hereby authorize and direct payment of the dental benefits otherwise payable to me, directly to the below named dentist or dental entity.

X_____
Subscriber signature   Date

BILLING DENTIST OR DENTAL ENTITY (Leave blank if dentist or dental entity is not submitting claim on behalf of the patient or insured/subscriber)

48. Name, Address, City, State, Zip Code

49. NPI	50. License Number	51. SSN or TIN

52. Phone Number ( ) –	52A. Additional Provider ID

ANCILLARY CLAIM/TREATMENT INFORMATION

38. Place of Treatment ☐ Provider's Office ☐ Hospital ☐ ECF ☐ Other	39. Number of Enclosures (00 to 99) Radiograph(s) Oral Image(s) Model(s)

40. Is Treatment for Orthodontics? ☐ No (Skip 41-42) ☐ Yes (Complete 41-42)	41. Date Appliance Placed (MM/DD/CCYY)

42. Months of Treatment Remaining	43. Replacement of Prosthesis? ☐ No ☐ Yes (Complete 44)	44. Date Prior Placement (MM/DD/CCYY)

45. Treatment Resulting from

☐ Occupational illness/injury ☐ Auto accident ☐ Other accident

46. Date of Accident (MM/DD/CCYY)	47. Auto Accident State

TREATING DENTIST AND TREATMENT LOCATION INFORMATION

53. I hereby certify that the procedures as indicated by date are in progress (for procedures that require multiple visits) or have been completed.

X_____
Signed (Treating Dentist)   Date

54. NPI	55. License Number

56. Address, City, State, Zip Code	56A. Provider Specialty Code

57. Phone Number ( ) –	58. Additional Provider ID

ADA. Dental Claim Form

HEADER INFORMATION

1. Type of Transaction (Mark all applicable boxes)

☐ Statement of Actual Services   ☐ Request for Predetermination/Preauthorization
☐ EPSDT/Title XIX

2. Predetermination/Preauthorization Number

INSURANCE COMPANY/DENTAL BENEFIT PLAN INFORMATION

3. Company/Plan Name, Address, City, State, Zip Code

OTHER COVERAGE

4. Other Dental or Medical Coverage?   ☐ No (Skip 5-11)   ☐ Yes (Complete 5-11)

5. Name of Policyholder/Subscriber in #4 (Last, First, Middle Initial, Suffix)

6. Date of Birth (MM/DD/CCYY)   7. Gender ☐ M ☐ F   8. Policyholder/Subscriber ID (SSN or ID#)

9. Plan/Group Number   10. Patient's Relationship to Person Named in #5
☐ Self ☐ Spouse ☐ Dependent ☐ Other

11. Other Insurance Company/Dental Benefit Plan Name, Address, City, State, Zip Code

POLICYHOLDER/SUBSCRIBER INFORMATION (For Insurance Company Named in #3)

12. Policyholder/Subscriber Name (Last, First, Middle Initial, Suffix), Address, City, State, Zip Code

13. Date of Birth (MM/DD/CCYY)   14. Gender ☐ M ☐ F   15. Policyholder/Subscriber ID (SSN or ID#)

16. Plan/Group Number   17. Employer Name

PATIENT INFORMATION

18. Relationship to Policyholder/Subscriber in #12 Above
☐ Self ☐ Spouse ☐ Dependent Child ☐ Other
19. Student Status ☐ FTS ☐ PTS

20. Name (Last, First, Middle Initial, Suffix), Address, City, State, Zip Code

21. Date of Birth (MM/DD/CCYY)   22. Gender ☐ M ☐ F   23. Patient ID/Account # (Assigned by Dentist)

RECORD OF SERVICES PROVIDED

	24. Procedure Date (MM/DD/CCYY)	25. Area of Oral Cavity	26. Tooth System	27. Tooth Number(s) or Letter(s)	28. Tooth Surface	29. Procedure Code	30. Description	31. Fee
1								
2								
3								
4								
5								
6								
7								
8								
9								
10								

MISSING TEETH INFORMATION

34. (Place an 'X' on each missing tooth)

Permanent: 1 2 3 4 5 6 7 8 9 10 11 12 13 14 15 16
32 31 30 29 28 27 26 25 24 23 22 21 20 19 18 17
Primary: A B C D E F G H I J
T S R Q P O N M L K

32. Other Fee(s)

33. Total Fee

35. Remarks

AUTHORIZATIONS

36. I have been informed of the treatment plan and associated fees. I agree to be responsible for all charges for dental services and materials not paid by my dental benefit plan, unless prohibited by law, or the treating dentist or dental practice has a contractual agreement with my plan prohibiting all or a portion of such charges. To the extent permitted by law, I consent to your use and disclosure of my protected health information to carry out payment activities in connection with this claim.

X _____
Patient/Guardian signature   Date

37. I hereby authorize and direct payment of the dental benefits otherwise payable to me, directly to the below named dentist or dental entity.

X _____
Subscriber signature   Date

BILLING DENTIST OR DENTAL ENTITY (Leave blank if dentist or dental entity is not submitting claim on behalf of the patient or insured/subscriber)

48. Name, Address, City, State, Zip Code

49. NPI   50. License Number   51. SSN or TIN

52. Phone Number ( )   –   52A. Additional Provider ID

ANCILLARY CLAIM/TREATMENT INFORMATION

38. Place of Treatment
☐ Provider's Office ☐ Hospital ☐ ECF ☐ Other

39. Number of Enclosures (00 to 99)
Radiograph(s) Oral Image(s) Model(s)

40. Is Treatment for Orthodontics?
☐ No (Skip 41-42) ☐ Yes (Complete 41-42)

41. Date Appliance Placed (MM/DD/CCYY)

42. Months of Treatment Remaining   43. Replacement of Prosthesis? ☐ No ☐ Yes (Complete 44)   44. Date Prior Placement (MM/DD/CCYY)

45. Treatment Resulting from
☐ Occupational illness/injury ☐ Auto accident ☐ Other accident

46. Date of Accident (MM/DD/CCYY)   47. Auto Accident State

TREATING DENTIST AND TREATMENT LOCATION INFORMATION

53. I hereby certify that the procedures as indicated by date are in progress (for procedures that require multiple visits) or have been completed.

X _____
Signed (Treating Dentist)   Date

54. NPI   55. License Number

56. Address, City, State, Zip Code   56A. Provider Specialty Code

57. Phone Number ( )   –   58. Additional Provider ID

©2006 American Dental Association
J400 (Same as ADA Dental Claim Form – J401, J402, J403, J404)

To Reorder call 1-800-947-4746
or go online at www.adacatalog.org

ADA. Dental Claim Form

HEADER INFORMATION

1. Type of Transaction (Mark all applicable boxes)

☐ Statement of Actual Services ☐ Request for Predetermination/Preauthorization

☐ EPSDT/Title XIX

2. Predetermination/Preauthorization Number

INSURANCE COMPANY/DENTAL BENEFIT PLAN INFORMATION

3. Company/Plan Name, Address, City, State, Zip Code

OTHER COVERAGE

4. Other Dental or Medical Coverage? ☐ No (Skip 5-11) ☐ Yes (Complete 5-11)

5. Name of Policyholder/Subscriber in #4 (Last, First, Middle Initial, Suffix)

6. Date of Birth (MM/DD/CCYY) | **7. Gender** ☐ M ☐ F | **8. Policyholder/Subscriber ID (SSN or ID#)**

9. Plan/Group Number | **10. Patient's Relationship to Person Named in #5** ☐ Self ☐ Spouse ☐ Dependent ☐ Other

11. Other Insurance Company/Dental Benefit Plan Name, Address, City, State, Zip Code

POLICYHOLDER/SUBSCRIBER INFORMATION (For Insurance Company Named in #3)

12. Policyholder/Subscriber Name (Last, First, Middle Initial, Suffix), Address, City, State, Zip Code

13. Date of Birth (MM/DD/CCYY) | **14. Gender** ☐ M ☐ F | **15. Policyholder/Subscriber ID (SSN or ID#)**

16. Plan/Group Number | **17. Employer Name**

PATIENT INFORMATION

18. Relationship to Policyholder/Subscriber in #12 Above ☐ Self ☐ Spouse ☐ Dependent Child ☐ Other | **19. Student Status** ☐ FTS ☐ PTS

20. Name (Last, First, Middle Initial, Suffix), Address, City, State, Zip Code

21. Date of Birth (MM/DD/CCYY) | **22. Gender** ☐ M ☐ F | **23. Patient ID/Account # (Assigned by Dentist)**

RECORD OF SERVICES PROVIDED

	24. Procedure Date (MM/DD/CCYY)	25. Area of Oral Cavity	26. Tooth System	27. Tooth Number(s) or Letter(s)	28. Tooth Surface	29. Procedure Code	30. Description	31. Fee
1								
2								
3								
4								
5								
6								
7								
8								
9								
10								

MISSING TEETH INFORMATION

34. (Place an 'X' on each missing tooth)

Permanent: 1 2 3 4 5 6 7 8 9 10 11 12 13 14 15 16 / 32 31 30 29 28 27 26 25 24 23 22 21 20 19 18 17

Primary: A B C D E F G H I J / T S R Q P O N M L K

32. Other Fee(s)

33. Total Fee

35. Remarks

AUTHORIZATIONS

36. I have been informed of the treatment plan and associated fees. I agree to be responsible for all charges for dental services and materials not paid by my dental benefit plan, unless prohibited by law, or the treating dentist or dental practice has a contractual agreement with my plan prohibiting all or a portion of such charges. To the extent permitted by law, I consent to your use and disclosure of my protected health information to carry out payment activities in connection with this claim.

X_____
Patient/Guardian signature   Date

37. I hereby authorize and direct payment of the dental benefits otherwise payable to me, directly to the below named dentist or dental entity.

X_____
Subscriber signature   Date

ANCILLARY CLAIM/TREATMENT INFORMATION

38. Place of Treatment ☐ Provider's Office ☐ Hospital ☐ ECF ☐ Other | **39. Number of Enclosures (00 to 99)** Radiograph(s) Oral Image(s) Model(s)

40. Is Treatment for Orthodontics? ☐ No (Skip 41-42) ☐ Yes (Complete 41-42) | **41. Date Appliance Placed (MM/DD/CCYY)**

42. Months of Treatment Remaining | **43. Replacement of Prosthesis?** ☐ No ☐ Yes (Complete 44) | **44. Date Prior Placement (MM/DD/CCYY)**

45. Treatment Resulting from ☐ Occupational illness/injury ☐ Auto accident ☐ Other accident

46. Date of Accident (MM/DD/CCYY) | **47. Auto Accident State**

BILLING DENTIST OR DENTAL ENTITY (Leave blank if dentist or dental entity is not submitting claim on behalf of the patient or insured/subscriber)

48. Name, Address, City, State, Zip Code

49. NPI | **50. License Number** | **51. SSN or TIN**

52. Phone Number ( ) – | **52A. Additional Provider ID**

TREATING DENTIST AND TREATMENT LOCATION INFORMATION

53. I hereby certify that the procedures as indicated by date are in progress (for procedures that require multiple visits) or have been completed.

X_____
Signed (Treating Dentist)   Date

54. NPI | **55. License Number**

56. Address, City, State, Zip Code | **56A. Provider Specialty Code**

57. Phone Number ( ) – | **58. Additional Provider ID**

Copyright © 2010. All rights reserved. Reprinted by permission. The ADA Claim Form is being revised in 2012 and may differ significantly from the current version printed in this publication.

For this exercise you will create a Dental Pretreatment Estimate. Please read the section in the Dentrix *User's Guide,* Family File, entitled "Creating a Dental Pretreatment Estimate" and complete the following patient-related forms:

19. Print a dental pretreatment estimate for Jana Rogers for the treatment of tooth #30.
    a. What is the total estimate charge?
    b. Did you include x-rays?
    c. What is the Dentrix code used for the root canal?
    d. What is listed in box #36?

Setting up and processing dental insurance with the aid of a practice management system is a very involved process. For a more in-depth description of the many functions that are available refer to the Dentrix *User's Guide,* Family File, section entitled "Working with Dental Insurance."

PUZZLE

Find the terms listed below. The first 30 letters not used in the puzzle will spell out a phrase.

Dental Insurance Processing

```
Y T D E N T A L I N F O E G S N U R A N C E P R O C S E E S
T N S S I N G T E E V E N R O M S V V K L X W R S L E N R U
R E O F S S A D E E F I F I V Q N C F W L Y P S A Q G C V P
A M L L L F U S R E L B T F H M W N W D B L K H F X R O H E
P Y F K C H C B L L C A B E N E F I T P A Y M E N T A U P R
D A A R L H I B I A Z V Y I N S U R E D R S D P V Q H N A B
R P Z G E L A B P I E R U T A L C N E M O N R E O K C T W I
I O P D L N E I R A U D I T E W C H E W Y E O O E A D E X L
H C U I O C T O W X J J W W R O A M K F C P P C R P E R G L
T L N S N A H E C I V R E S T I F E N E B D D N T P R F N S
E G A A T T A N W F U C M S E W O K R D T E U D E Y E O I J
S E L I U E W A N U I S W U U F F T T D P X I E E O V R D E
R A O A F K U U T V N O I T A N I M R E T E D E R P O M O T
B N E P M A E T R G R U F R B F O Y N T E R E R U K C S C U
S R P O E N T E X P I R A T I O N D A T E O A F E M O Z N S
P B U N G N S E F U E O L C C U E X C X S T F K L Y T T W L
V W S S S R E E L L K R A E U N X J C E T A A M L A A X O X
A W R R O U T N E B O T S N T G E N D E R R U L E S U P D X
D T T F U B U B R F I E T S A H S Y O D A T S T N P T S T L
E T E R T T T W T O F T R U W L E B X C T S P T A U R T U X
R E R R H S N T N T L O C A U L E B F C U I O W P T R X T C
F S N O I S U L C X E L G U C O F B C F X N O X D U T I C Z
E L U R Y A D H T R I B M N D D J A B B A I J X E M T N K H
C R E B I R C S B U S C D E I E E F Y R A M O T S U C S R U
L E N A P N E P O F F E L A N L D G F F X D J P O T T U C K
F K M A E T M R H A N K Y A T T I F A F R A A O L E T R K O
N A L P Y T I N M E D N I H I F F F R N R X R S C E T E R V
O V E R C O D I N G A O N G Y M R R E R A R J L F R F R H D
B L S O D G B K B A F J T T W Y N K Y R R M A E F O F T O M
W F B S E G R A H C E L B A W O L L A I P I R R O Y F K M A
```

ADMINISTRATOR	GENDER RULE
ALLOWABLE CHARGES	INDEMNITY PLAN
AUDIT	INSURED
BALANCE BILLING	INSURER
BENEFIT PAYMENT	MANAGED CARE
BENEFIT SERVICE	NOMENCLATURE
BIRTHDAY RULE	OPEN ENROLLMENT
CAPITATION	OPEN PANEL
CLAIM	OVERBILLING
CLOSED PANEL	OVERCODING
COPAYMENT	PAYER
COVERED CHARGES	PREAUTHORIZATION
CUSTOMARY FEE	PRECERTIFICATION
DEDUCTIBLE	PREDETERMINATION
DEPENDENTS	PREFILING OF FEES
DOWNCODING	REASONABLE FEE
ENCOUNTER FORMS	SUBSCRIBER
EXCLUSIONS	SUPERBILLS
EXPIRATION DATE	THIRD PARTY
FEE FOR SERVICE	USUAL FEE
FEE SCHEDULE	

16 Bookkeeping Procedures: Accounts Payable

INTRODUCTION

Accounts payable is a system in which all of the dental practice expenditures are organized, verified, and categorized. The system identifies when checks for bills (including payroll) are to be written, verifies charges, and categorizes expenditures. Other elements of the accounts payable system include reconciliation of the checking accounts and preparation of documents for the accountant.

LEARNING OBJECTIVES

1. Describe the function of accounts payable.
2. Formulate a system by which to organize accounts payable.
3. Analyze the methods of check writing and state their functions.
4. Discuss steps to follow to reconcile a checking account and list the necessary information.
5. List and discuss the information needed for a payroll record.

EXERCISES

1. Describe the function of accounts payable.

2. List the four ways checks can be written.

3. List the steps involved in writing a check.

4. List the information needed for a payroll record.

_____

_____

_____

_____

_____

_____

_____

_____

ACTIVITY EXERCISE

For the following exercises, you will be calculating payroll, writing checks, balancing the checkbook, and reconciling the bank statement. It is important to work through this exercise sequentially because information needed will be obtained from completed exercises and forms.

Scenario: Your assignment today as the administrative dental assistant is to calculate the payroll, pay bills, balance the checkbook, and reconcile the bank statement.

5. Total the hours worked for Sue Smith:
   Time Card
   Employee: Sue Smith
   Pay period: 4/1 to 4/13

Date	Time in	Time out	Time in	Time out	Total hours
4/1	8:00	12:00	1:30	5:30	
4/2	8:15	12:00	1:00	5:00	
4/3	10:00	1:00	2:00	6:00	
4/5	7:45	12:15	1:30	5:00	
4/6	7:30	1:30			
4/9	8:00	12:00	1:30	5:30	
4/10	8:00	12:00	1:00	5:00	
4/11	10:00	1:00	2:00	6:00	
4/12	7:45	12:15	1:30	5:00	
4/13	7:30	1:30			
				TOTAL HOURS WORKED	

6. Refer to Sue's payroll record (see p. 105) for the following information:
   Marital Status _____
   Exemptions _____
   Rate of Pay _____

7. Calculate the following for Sue Smith:
   Gross Salary (Refer to Sue's payroll record and the time card to calculate.) $ _____
   Federal Withholding
   (See Tax Table on the following page.) $ _____
   FICA Tax (6.2%) $ _____
   Medicare (1.45%) $ _____
   Pension (6%) $ _____

8. Refer to Edith's payroll record (p. 105) for the following information:
   Marital Status   _____
   Exemptions   _____
   Rate of Pay   _____

9. Calculate the following for Edith Gates:
   Gross Salary (Refer to Edith's payroll record to calculate) $ _____
   Federal Withholding
   (See Tax Table on the following page.) $ _____
   FICA Tax (6.2%) $ _____
   Medicare (1.45%) $ _____
   Pension (6%) $ _____

Date all checks 4/13 of the current year.

MARRIED Persons—SEMIMONTHLY Payroll Period

(For Wages Paid through December 2011)

And the wages are—		And the number of withholding allowances claimed is—										
At least	But less than	0	1	2	3	4	5	6	7	8	9	10
		The amount of income tax to be withheld is—										
$1,500	$1,520	$142	$119	$95	$72	$56	$41	$26	$10	$0	$0	$0
1,520	1,540	145	122	98	75	58	43	28	12	0	0	0
1,540	1,560	148	125	101	78	60	45	30	14	0	0	0
1,560	1,580	151	128	104	81	62	47	32	16	1	0	0
1,580	1,600	154	131	107	84	64	49	34	18	3	0	0
1,600	1,620	157	134	110	87	66	51	36	20	5	0	0
1,620	1,640	160	137	113	90	68	53	38	22	7	0	0
1,640	1,660	163	140	116	93	70	55	40	24	9	0	0
1,660	1,680	166	143	119	96	73	57	42	26	11	0	0
1,680	1,700	169	146	122	99	76	59	44	28	13	0	0
1,700	1,720	172	149	125	102	79	61	46	30	15	0	0
1,720	1,740	175	152	128	105	82	63	48	32	17	1	0
1,740	1,760	178	155	131	108	85	65	50	34	19	3	0
1,760	1,780	181	158	134	111	88	67	52	36	21	5	0
1,780	1,800	184	161	137	114	91	69	54	38	23	7	0
1,800	1,820	187	164	140	117	94	71	56	40	25	9	0
1,820	1,840	190	167	143	120	97	74	58	42	27	11	0
1,840	1,860	193	170	146	123	100	77	60	44	29	13	0
1,860	1,880	196	173	149	126	103	80	62	46	31	15	0
1,880	1,900	199	176	152	129	106	83	64	48	33	17	2
1,900	1,920	202	179	155	132	109	86	66	50	35	19	4
1,920	1,940	205	182	158	135	112	89	68	52	37	21	6
1,940	1,960	208	185	161	138	115	92	70	54	39	23	8
1,960	1,980	211	188	164	141	118	95	72	56	41	25	10
1,980	2,000	214	191	167	144	121	98	75	58	43	27	12
2,000	2,020	217	194	170	147	124	101	78	60	45	29	14
2,020	2,040	220	197	173	150	127	104	81	62	47	31	16
2,040	2,060	223	200	176	153	130	107	84	64	49	33	18
2,060	2,080	226	203	179	156	133	110	87	66	51	35	20
2,080	2,100	229	206	182	159	136	113	90	68	53	37	22
2,100	2,120	232	209	185	162	139	116	93	70	55	39	24
2,120	2,140	235	212	188	165	142	119	96	73	57	41	26
2,140	2,160	238	215	191	168	145	122	99	76	59	43	28
2,160	2,180	241	218	194	171	148	125	102	79	61	45	30
2,180	2,200	244	221	197	174	151	128	105	82	63	47	32
2,200	2,220	247	224	200	177	154	131	108	85	65	49	34
2,220	2,240	250	227	203	180	157	134	111	88	67	51	36
2,240	2,260	253	230	206	183	160	137	114	91	69	53	38
2,260	2,280	256	233	209	186	163	140	117	94	71	55	40
2,280	2,300	259	236	212	189	166	143	120	97	74	57	42
2,300	2,320	262	239	215	192	169	146	123	100	77	59	44
2,320	2,340	265	242	218	195	172	149	126	103	80	61	46
2,340	2,360	268	245	221	198	175	152	129	106	83	63	48
2,360	2,380	271	248	224	201	178	155	132	109	86	65	50
2,380	2,400	274	251	227	204	181	158	135	112	89	67	52
2,400	2,420	277	254	230	207	184	161	138	115	92	69	54
2,420	2,440	280	257	233	210	187	164	141	118	95	72	56
2,440	2,460	283	260	236	213	190	167	144	121	98	75	58
2,460	2,480	286	263	239	216	193	170	147	124	101	78	60
2,480	2,500	289	266	242	219	196	173	150	127	104	81	62
2,500	2,520	292	269	245	222	199	176	153	130	107	84	64
2,520	2,540	295	272	248	225	202	179	156	133	110	87	66
2,540	2,560	298	275	251	228	205	182	159	136	113	90	68
2,560	2,580	301	278	254	231	208	185	162	139	116	93	70
2,580	2,600	304	281	257	234	211	188	165	142	119	96	72
2,600	2,620	307	284	260	237	214	191	168	145	122	99	75
2,620	2,640	310	287	263	240	217	194	171	148	125	102	78
2,640	2,660	313	290	266	243	220	197	174	151	128	105	81
2,660	2,680	316	293	269	246	223	200	177	154	131	108	84
2,680	2,700	319	296	272	249	226	203	180	157	134	111	87
2,700	2,720	322	299	275	252	229	206	183	160	137	114	90
2,720	2,740	325	302	278	255	232	209	186	163	140	117	93

$2,740 and over	Use Table 3(b) for a **MARRIED person** on page 36. Also see the instructions on page 35.

10. Using information from Question 7, complete the following payroll record for Sue Smith:

Marital status **M** _____
Number of Exp **1** _____

EMPLOYEE'S PAYROLL RECORD

Name: **Sue Smith** _____ Social Security Number: **620-31-8752** _____

Address: **18 N. Fox Glenn** _____ City: **CanyonView** _____ Zip code _____

Telephone:**555-3816** _____ Date of Birth: **06/20/70** _____

Occupation: **Dental Assistant** _____ Date of employment: **10/2** _____

Pay rate: **$19.50** _____

	Date	Check number	Gross salary	Fed W/H	FICA	M/C	State W/H	Other	Net check
	Total								

11. Write a payroll check for Ms. Smith.

Mary A. Edwards, D.D.S.
4546 North Avery Way
Canyon View, CA 91783

YOUR BANK HERE
CITY, STATE ZIP

00-0000
0000

No. 3223

PAY _____ DOLLARS

TO THE
ORDER OF _____

DISC.	DATE	CHECK NO.	AMOUNT	
			DOLLARS	CTS.

YOUR NAME HERE

⑈00 18 54⑈ ⑉000000000⑉ 00000000⑈

12. Using information from Question 9, complete the following payroll record for Edith Gates:

Marital status **M** _____
Number of Exp **3** _____

EMPLOYEE'S PAYROLL RECORD

Name: **Edith Gates** _____ Social Security Number: **608-31-8211** _____

Address: **46472 5th St.** _____ City: **Canyon View** _____ Zip code _____

Telephone:**555-0182** _____ Date of Birth: **10/18/46** _____

Occupation: **Insurance Clerk** _____ Date of employment: _____

Pay rate: **$1800.00 Semimonthly** _____

	Date	Check number	Gross salary	Fed W/H	FICA	M/C	State W/H	Other	Net check
	Total								

Chapter **16** Bookkeeping Procedures: Accounts Payable

13. Write a payroll check for Ms. Gates.

Mary A. Edwards, D.D.S.
4546 North Avery Way
Canyon View, CA 91783

YOUR BANK HERE
CITY, STATE ZIP

00-0000
0000

No. 3224

PAY _____ DOLLARS

TO THE
ORDER OF _____

DISC.	DATE	CHECK NO.	AMOUNT	
			DOLLARS	CTS.

YOUR NAME HERE

⑈OO 18 54⑈ ⑈OOOOOOOOO⑈ OOOOOOOO⑈

14. Pay an invoice in the amount of $32.46 for the postcards you ordered. Make the check payable to Speedy Stationery Supplies.

Mary A. Edwards, D.D.S.
4546 North Avery Way
Canyon View, CA 91783

YOUR BANK HERE
CITY, STATE ZIP

00-0000
0000

No. 3225

PAY _____ DOLLARS

TO THE
ORDER OF _____

DISC.	DATE	CHECK NO.	AMOUNT	
			DOLLARS	CTS.

YOUR NAME HERE

⑈OO 18 54⑈ ⑈OOOOOOOOO⑈ OOOOOOOO⑈

15. Pay the invoice from City Insurance Services in the amount of $910.00 for professional insurance.

Mary A. Edwards, D.D.S.
4546 North Avery Way
Canyon View, CA 91783

YOUR BANK HERE
CITY, STATE ZIP

00-0000
0000

No. 3226

PAY _____ DOLLARS

TO THE
ORDER OF _____

DISC.	DATE	CHECK NO.	AMOUNT	
			DOLLARS	CTS.

YOUR NAME HERE

⑈OO 18 54⑈ ⑈OOOOOOOOO⑈ OOOOOOOO⑈

16. Record the checks you have just written in the following checkbook register:

MONTH April
PAGE 1

CHECK REGISTER

#	PAID TO	DISC.	DATE	CHECK NUMBER	AMOUNT		EXPLANATION	BANK BALANCE	BANK DEPOSIT AMOUNT		DATE
	BALANCE FORWARDED				-0-			5,322 13			
1	Smith Labs		4/1	3215	482	31	lab		4231	00	4/1
2	Diane Blangsted		4/1	3216	1827	75	payroll		2383	00	4/2
3	Dianna Rogers		4/1	3217	331	06	payroll		3892	00	4/3
4	ABC Dental Supplies		4/1	3218	318	00	supplies		2341	00	4/8
5	Edison		4/1	3219	212	46	utility		23	00	4/10
6	Phone Company		4/1	3220	281	12	utility				
7	Dental Lab Inc.	hh	4/1	3221	892	00	lab				
8	Payroll Tax		4/1	3222	400	00	prof tax				
9	Office Rental		4/1	electronic	2122	00	rent				
10	Postage		4/1	Phone order debit card	216	00	stamps				
11											
12											
13											
14											
15											
16											
17											
18											
19											
20											
21											
22											
23											
24											
	TOTALS (THIS PAGE)										
	TOTALS MONTH TO DATE										
	TOTALS YEAR TO DATE										

Chapter **16** **Bookkeeping Procedures: Accounts Payable**

17. Record the following deposit information for 4/12.
Cash: $187.00
Checks: $852.00
Total: deposit $1,039.00
Total credit card deposit: $2,442.00

18. Balance the checkbook register (Question 16) by adding all columns. (Remember Before adding the columns, enter the checks you have written in Questions 11, 13, 14, and 15 and the deposits in question 17.)
Answer the following questions:
Total of all checks/debits this page $ _____
Total deposits/credits $ _____
Beginning balance $ _____

19. Calculate checkbook balance. (Use information from the checkbook register in Question 16.)
Beginning balance $ _____
Add bank deposits/credits $ _____
Subtotal $ _____
Less total checks/debits $ _____
New bank balance $ _____

It is the end of the month, and you have received the bank statement. Your assignment is to reconcile the checkbook. After checking for outstanding checks and deposits in transit, you identify the following information as outstanding:

Check numbers	3190	$ 11.86	
	3210	$103.24	
	3219	$221.46	
Deposit			$2,442.00
Current statements ending balance		$9,033.23	

20. Complete the following worksheet:

BALANCING YOUR CHECKBOOK
Worksheet

STEP 1
List all deposits and all credits that do not appear on the bank statement

STEP 2
List outstanding checks, withdrawals and other debits that do not appear on the bank statement

Date	Amount		Check #	Amount	
Total	$		**Total**	$	

Calculation worksheet

CURRENT STATEMENT'S ENDING BALANCE	$	
Add deposits/other credits not yet credited on this statement (Step 1) +	$	
SUBTOTAL =	$	
Subtract checks/other debits not listed on this statement (Step 2) −	$	
CURRENT CHECKBOOK BALANCE =	$	

21. What are the total deposits that do not appear on the bank statement? $_____

22. What is the total of outstanding checks? $_____

23. What is the current checkbook balance from the worksheet? $_____

24. What is the current checkbook balance from the checkbook register? $_____

25. Do the current checkbook balance (from the checkbook register in question 16) and the balance from the worksheet match? If not, find your error.

Using the clues below, fill in the crossword puzzle.

Accounts Payable

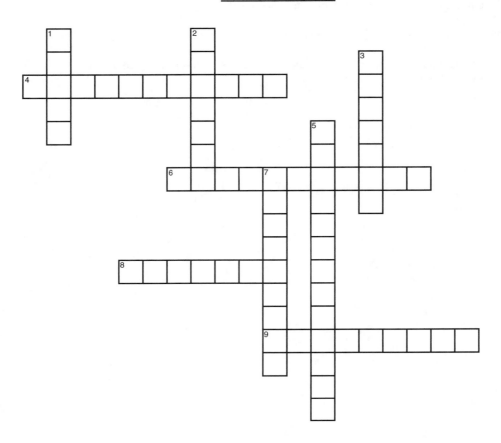

Across

4. Method used to ensure that practice and bank records are in agreement
6. Identifies the account and includes amount of money being deposited
8. List of purchased items and their charges
9. Amount of money given an employee after deductions

Down

1. Paper method of remitting payment
2. Amount of money available after all deposits and checks have been recorded
3. Method for issuing money to employees
5. Remitting payment via telephone and computerized online service, and automatic payments
7. List of the totals of all invoices

17 Bookkeeping Procedures: Accounts Receivable

INTRODUCTION

Dentistry, like any business, is mandated by federal and state regulations to maintain a system that documents the collection of monies. Smart business practice also requires maintenance of a financial system that includes both accounts receivable and accounts payable. It is the responsibility of the administrative dental assistant to maintain accurate records in the management of accounts receivable and accounts payable.

LEARNING OBJECTIVES

1. Discuss the role of the administrative dental assistant in the management of patient financial transactions.
2. Describe the steps in posting transactions: charges, payments and adjustments, and proof of posting.
3. Discuss the importance of an audit report.
4. Describe a process for implementing an audit trail. Compare the audit trails used in a computerized with those used in a manual bookkeeping system.

EXERCISES

1. Describe the role of the administrative dental assistant in managing patient financial transactions.

_____

_____

_____

_____

2. List and define the components of a pegboard bookkeeping system.

_____

_____

_____

3. Describe the purpose of an audit report.

_____

_____

4. List two reasons why audit reports are necessary.

_____

_____

5. List the five steps to be followed in completing an audit report.

_____

_____

_____

_____

_____

ACTIVITY EXERCISE

For this exercise, you will need your clinical records for

    Jana Rogers

    Holly Barry

    Angelica Green

    Lynn Bacca

Remember: You will find the information you will need to complete this assignment on the **Treatment Plan Form** and **Financial Arrangement Form.**

Scenario

Today is April 12. You are completing your task of posting transactions for the day. You need to post transactions for your last four patients: Jana Rogers, Angelica Green, Holly Barry, and Lynn Bacca. When you have posted these transactions, it will be time to perform the end-of-day function of balancing the day sheet.

6. Use the Daily Log of Charges and Receipts on p. 114 to perform the following functions:
    A. Post transactions on the Daily Log for Jana Rogers, Angelica Green, Holly Barry, and Lynn Bacca using the following information and information from their clinical records (treatments for April 12 and financial arrangements).
    B. Complete the end-of-day procedure by totaling all columns and completing the proof of posting.

Posting Information

Jana Rogers
    Previous Balance $000.00
    Payment (cash) .... $ 75.00
Angelica Green
    Previous Balance $125.00
    Payment $000.00
Holly Barry
    Previous Balance $125.00
    Payment (credit card) .... per financial agreement
    Senior Citizen Discount .... per financial agreement
Lynn Bacca
    Previous Balance $000.00
    Payment (cash) .... $ 50.00

Complete the following using information from the Daily Log (p. 114).

7. Proof of posting

Column D total .... $_____
Plus Column A total .... $_____
Subtotal .... $_____
Less Columns B1 & B2 .... $_____
Must equal Column C .... $_____

8. Accounts receivable control

Previous day's total .... $ 1098.10
Plus Column A total .... $_____
Subtotal .... $_____
Less Columns B1 & B2 .... $_____
Total accounts receivable .... $_____

9. Accounts receivable proof

Accts receivable 1st of month .... $ 0000.00
Plus Column A month to date .... $_____
Subtotal .... $_____
Less Columns B1 & B2 mo. to date .... $_____
Total accounts receivable .... $_____

115

DAILY LOG OF CHARGES AND RECEIPTS

DATE __4/12__ SHEET NUMBER _____ A B1 B2 C D

	DATE	FAMILY MEMBER	PROFESSIONAL SERVICES	CHARGE	CREDITS		NEW BALANCE	PREVIOUS BALANCE	NAME
					PYMTS.	ADJ			
1	4/12	Rose	ins. pmt./adj.		98 00	12 00	80 00	190 00	Rose Budd
2	4/12	Frank	NSF	80 00	—	—	80 00	-0-	Frank Williams
3	4/12	Judy	payment	—	62 00	—	<22 00>	40 00	Judy Coulson
4	4/12	Dawn	Restorative	230 00	-0-	—	240 00	10 00	Dawn Johnson
5	4/12	Maria	prophy/c.pmt.	62 00	62 00	—	-0-	-0-	Marie Gonzales
6	4/12	Angela	FMX	80 00	62 00	—	80 00	62 00	Angela Brown
7	4/12	Mark	Composite	246 00	—	24 60	221 40	-0-	Mark Vail
8	4/12	Lois	ins. pmt.	—	630 00	20 00	171 00	821 00	Lois Tracy
9									
10									
11									
12									
13									
14									
15									
16									
17									
18									
19									
20									
21									
22									
23									
24									
25									
26									
27									
28									
29									
30									
31									
32									

TOTALS — THIS PAGE / PREVIOUS PAGE / MONTH-TO-DATE

3240 00	2163 00	<21 10>	5419 10	4321 00
Col. "A"	Col. "B-1"	Col. "B-2"	Col. "C"	Col. "D"

DENTRIX EXERCISE*

As part of the daily routine you will perform a series of tasks that will organize the day, track patient treatment, post patient transactions, check out a patient, and schedule new appointments.

Before you can complete the following tasks, it will be necessary to move the patients you scheduled during the Dentrix Appointment Book exercise to the current day.

Moving Appointments

Whether a patient needs to reschedule or the office needs to lighten the schedule, from time to time you will need to move an already scheduled appointment to a new date or time. You can either move an appointment directly to a new date and time or move it temporarily to the Pinboard. *Note:* You can move appointments in Day View and Week View but not in Month View.

*Dentrix exercises based on content and screen captures courtesy Henry Schein Practice Solutions, American Fork, Utah.

Moving an Appointment Directly to a New Date and Time

1. Set the Day View or Week View, depending on whether you are moving the appointment to a different time in the same day or to a different day of the same week.

2. In Appointment Book, click the appointment that you want to move and drag it to the new date.

3. When the **Move Appointment** message appears, click **Yes**.

Moving an Appointment to the Pinboard

1. In the Appointment Book, click the appointment that you want to move and drag it to the Pinboard in the upper right corner of the Appointment Book.

2. Find a new date and time for the appointment.

3. Click the appointment icon on the Pinboard and drag the appointment to the new date and time.

4. When the Move appointment message appears, click **Yes.**
   Tip: If you know the exact date and time to which you want to move an appointment, double click the appointment to open the **Appointment Information** dialog box, enter the new date and time in the date and time field and click **OK**.

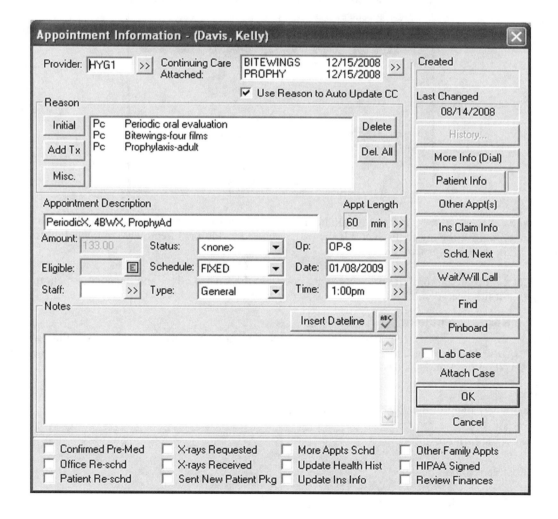

Chapter **17** Bookkeeping Procedures: Accounts Receivable

Route Slips

The Dentrix Route Slip can be used for a variety of information purposes: as a reminder of Medical Alerts, for patient notes, and for collection information for patients being seen that day. Also, all future appointments for every family member appear on the Patient Route Slip. (Dentrix now offers a customizable type or route slip called the Patient Visit Form. See the *User's Guide* for more detailed information.) To generate a route slip:

1. From the Appointment Book, select an appointment.

2. From the Appointment Book toolbar, click the **Print Route Slip** button. The Print Route Slip dialog box appears.

3. To print the report immediately, click the **Print** button.

Posting Scheduled Work

Once an appointment has been completed, you can quickly post procedures attached to the appointment with the click of one button. To post appointment procedures:

1. In the Appointment Book, select the Appointment you want to post complete.

2. From the Appointment Book toolbar, click the **Set Complete** button. The Set Appointment Procedure Complete dialog box appears.

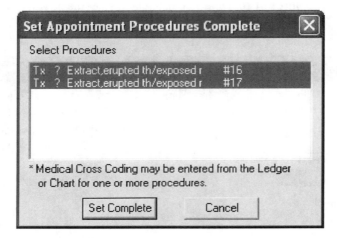

1. All procedures attached to the appointment are highlighted. If a procedure has not been completed on this visit, click it once to remove the highlight. *Note:* If the patient has had additional treatment completed during the visit, post the work in the Chart or Ledger.

2. Click the **Set Complete** button. The procedures are posted to the Chart/Ledger and the appointment turns gray, indicating that it has been completed.

Scheduling the Next Appointment

For detailed directions refer to the Dentrix *User's Guide*, Appointment Book, section entitled "Scheduling Appointments." (*Note:* The Dentrix *User's Guide* is provided in electronic format on the Dentrix Learning Edition DVD and also saved on the Windows desktop when the Learning Edition is installed.)

Scheduling Tips

1. Right click on the patient in the Appointment Book (notice all of the options).

2. Click, **Other Appointments**.

3. Select the treatment to be scheduled.

4. Click **Create New Appt.**

5. Complete the **Appointment Information** dialog box. (See the Dentrix *User's Guide* for detailed instructions.)

Fast Checkout Button

When a patient checks out of the dental office, three tasks can be completed with the click of a button. The **Fast Checkout** button, located on the Ledger toolbar, allows you to quickly post a payment, generate an insurance claim, and print a receipt. You can customize the **Fast Checkout** button to meet the needs of the office. For this exercise, set the following options:

1. Select **File**, then **Fast Checkout Options Setup**. The Fast Checkout Options Setup dialog box appears.

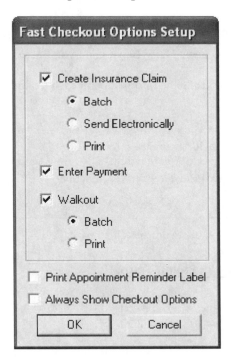

2. Set up the following tasks:
   a. Click **Create Insurance Claim;** then select **Print.**
   b. Click **Enter Payment.**
   c. Click **Walkout,** and then select **Print.**
   d. Click **Always show Checkout options.**
   e. Click **OK.**

Using Fast Checkout

1. Click the **Select Patient** button on the Ledger toolbar.

2. If you have not already posted the procedures for this patient, post them at this time.

3. From the Ledger toolbar, click the **Fast Checkout** button. If you have set the button option to always show Checkout Options, the Checkout Options Setup dialog box appears.

4. Select the desired option(s) if necessary.

5. Click **OK.**

6. The Enter Payment dialog box appears. Enter the payment information and click **OK.**

Chapter **17** **Bookkeeping Procedures: Accounts Receivable**

Patient Exercises

Scenario: As part of your daily routine, print out a copy of the Appointment Book for each operatory and a route slip for the patients you have scheduled (Jana Rogers, Angelica Green, Holly Barry, and Lynn Bacca). At the end of each appointment, check out the patient by posting scheduled work, scheduling the next appointment, posting payments, and printing an insurance claim and walkout statement.

At the end of this exercise you will have

1. Printed a copy of the Appointment Book view

2. Generated route slips for Jana Rogers, Angelica Green, Holly Barry, and Lynn Bacca

3. Scheduled the next appointment for each patient, using the information in each treatment plan

4. Collected payments

5. Printed an insurance claim form for each patient with insurance information

6. Printed a walkout statement (Statement of Services Rendered) for each patient

PUZZLE

Search for the **BOLDFACE CAPITALIZED** terms in this word search puzzle.

Bookkeeping Terms

```
L A K W R H I E A Q T M H I D M K E S G
C S L S P E O C Z Y Q P O J P J L O N J
C Y C L P G C O A A N Q V O D B O I J F
Q L Z V S I T E G V K R R W A R T P R B
O I R C A K L A I U K O Y V N N N E Y L
T W H R P C V S N P F Y I H U D E G E W
U M X Y X H C Y G P T E L O T V K B K L
N J R H E Z G O P N C S C L G O P O Q G
Y F J Q N R B O U E I C T T O W B A S G
C I V J P M S P R N A T K L G O B R G N
Y N J D D T O S Q N T T U T D W I D H I
B Y S N I S T F R S Y S G O H Q Y S A P
A F I N A N C I A L R E P O R T S Y T E
B Q G K U G D A T T V K N A B K G S H E
C T L O N D J P M M A S B D Y J E T H K
S Y C T X X H C D X M F U C V A Q E N K
F C T H O M B A J G M F W P B S B M R O
A N N X S C C H A R G E S L I P E L C O
L A N R U O J Y L I A D Z A M G S K E B
S U T S Y T X C H H A Z G B Y O M K W E
```

ACCOUNTING

ACCOUNTS PAYABLE

ACCOUNTS RECEIVABLE

AGING

BOOKKEEPING

CHARGE SLIP

DAILY JOURNAL

FINANCIAL REPORTS

PEGBOARD SYSTEM

POSTING Transactions

RECEIPTS

ROUTING SLIPS

18 Employment Strategies

INTRODUCTION

Hundreds of jobs are waiting for the right people to fill them. The hiring decision is based on the ability of the prospective employee to successfully present himself or herself. Convincing the employer that you are the best person for the job is not easy. The process begins with a self-study and ends with a personal interview. Along the way, you will identify career options, answer questions about yourself, research possible employment opportunities, and produce a quality resume. You will also construct a letter of introduction, complete an application, and prepare mentally and physically for an interview.

LEARNING OBJECTIVES

1. List the career opportunities for administrative dental assistants.
2. Identify the steps to be followed in developing an employment strategy. Discuss the function of each step.
3. Produce a quality resume.
4. Write a cover letter.
5. Explain the function of a personal career portfolio and discuss its advantages.
6. Plan a personal employment strategy.

EXERCISES

1. List the career opportunities for an administrative dental assistant.

_____

_____

_____

_____

_____

2. List and state the purpose of the steps involved in developing employment strategies.

_____

_____

_____

_____

_____

_____

_____

3. Describe the function of a personal career portfolio.

_____

_____

_____

_____

4. List the components of a personal career portfolio.

_____

_____

_____

_____

_____

5. List the components of a quality resume.

_____

_____

_____

_____

_____

6. List the various avenues that may lead to employment.

_____

_____

_____

_____

_____

_____

7. Select a resume style (a chronological resume, a functional resume, or a hybrid resume) and produce a high-quality resume.

8. Write a cover letter.

PUZZLE

Unscramble each of the clue words. Take the letters in the numbered cells and match them with cells with the same number in the boxes underneath the clue words.

Resumes

CIAGOCNLORLOH RSMEUE

VEORC TERTEL

NAOTIDAECLU SIENUTTIST

LAUFONNICT SEMREU

HIYRDB MUSERE

JBO CASHER LGO

CIBTEJOEV

RPSEOLAN RARECE TOLPORFOI

SOIRELFOSNAP NAORIGSATNOZI

Appendix: Patient Paperwork

All forms in this appendix courtesy The Dental Record, Wisconsin Dental Association, Milwaukee, WI.

Jana Rogers

welcome

| | | | | | | | |

PATIENT NUMBER

© 2003 Wisconsin Dental Association
(800) 243-4675

Date _____

Patient's Name _____
Last   First   Initial

Date of Birth _____ ❑ Male ❑ Female

If Child: Parent's Name _____

How do you wish to be addressed _____
Single ❑ Married ❑ Separated ❑ Divorced ❑ Widowed ❑ Minor ❑

Residence - Street _____

City _____ State _____ Zip _____

Business Address _____

Telephone: Res. _____ Bus. _____

Fax _____ Cell Phone # _____

eMail _____

Patient/Parent Employed By _____

Present Position _____

How Long Held _____

Spouse/Parent Name _____

Spouse Employed By _____

Present Position _____

How Long Held _____

Who is Responsible for this account _____

Drivers License No. _____

Method of Payment: Insurance ❑ Cash ❑ Credit Card ❑

Purpose of Call _____

Other Family Members in this Practice _____

_____

Whom may we thank for this referral _____

Patient/parent Social Security No. _____

Spouse/Parent Social Security No. _____

Someone to notify in case of emergency not living with you _____

DENTAL INSURANCE 1ST COVERAGE

Employee Name _____ Date of Birth _____
Employer Name _____ Yrs. _____
Name of Insurance Co. _____
Address _____
_____
Telephone _____
Program or policy # _____
Social Security No. _____
Union Local or Group _____

DENTAL INSURANCE 2ND COVERAGE

Employee Name _____ Date of Birth _____
Employer Name _____ Yrs. _____
Name of Insurance Co. _____
Address _____
_____
Telephone _____
Program or policy # _____
Social Security No. _____
Union Local or Group _____

CONSENT:
I consent to the diagnostic procedures and treatment by the dentist necessary for proper dental care.

I consent to the dentist's use and disclosure of my records (or my child's records) to carry out treatment, to obtain payment, and for those activities and health care operations that are related to treatment or payment.

I consent to the disclosure of my records (or my child's records) to the following persons who are involved in my care (or my child's care) or payment for that care.

_____

My consent to disclosure of records shall be effective until I revoke it in writing.

I authorize payment directly to the dentist or dental group of insurance benefits otherwise payable to me. I understand that my dental care insurance carrier or payor of my dental benefits may pay less than the actual bill for services, and that I am financially responsible for payment in full of all accounts. By signing this statement, I revoke all previous agreements to the contrary and agree to be responsible for payment of services not paid, by my dental care payor.

I attest to the accuracy of the information on this page.

PATIENT'S OR GUARDIAN'S SIGNATURE

_____

DATE _____

Form No. T110R

REGISTRATION

Jana Rogers

× | PATIENT NUMBER | ×

PATIENT'S NAME _____
Last   First   Initial

RHEUMATIC FEVER	ALLERGIES	AIDS	HEPATITIS	HEART COND.	MEDICATION	ANESTHETIC	BLOOD PRESSURE	PULSE

MISSING TEETH & EXISTING RESTORATIONS

1 2 3 4 5 6 7 8   9 10 11 12 13 14 15 16

B

L
DATE _____
RIGHT

A B C D E   F G H I J
T S R Q P   O N M L K   LEFT

L

B

32 31 30 29 28 27 26 25   24 23 22 21 20 19 18 17

PATIENT'S CHIEF COMPLAINT:

EXISTING X-RAYS   DATE

BW _____
PAN _____
FMX _____
PA _____

PROSTHESIS EVALUATION
TYPE OR AREA   DATE INSERTED

SOFT TISSUE EXAMINATION	OK

COMMENTS:

OCCLUSION   EVALUATION

TMJ EVALUATION

Right: n Crepitus   n Snapping/Popping
Left: n Crepitus   n Snapping/Popping

Tenderness to Palpation:
TMJ: n Right   n Left
Muscles: _____
Deviation on Closing: ____Rmm_____Lmm
Maximum Opening: _____ mm

COMMENTS:

CONDITIONS / TREATMENT INDICATED

1 2 3 4 5 6 7 8   9 10 11 12 13 14 15 16

B

L
DATE _____
RIGHT

A B C D E   F G H I J
T S R Q P   O N M L K   LEFT

L

B

32 31 30 29 28 27 26 25   24 23 22 21 20 19 18 17

Treatment Schedule n

SIGNATURE OF DENTIST

CLINICAL EXAMINATION

Form No. T170CE

Jana Rogers

PATIENT NUMBER

PATIENT'S NAME _____

Last   First   Initial   Date

DATE	TREATMENT PLAN	FEE	ALTERNATE TREATMENT	FEE	PROB # ASGN

RELEASE:

I accept the above treatment plan. I understand that because of unexpected circumstances, the treatment, the fees for treatment and/or the materials required as explained to me at this time, may require some changes after actual care has begun.

PATIENT'S/GUARDIAN'S SIGNATURE _____ DATE _____

| ANEST. |

| MED. ALERT |

Form No. T201TP

TREATMENT PLAN

Jana Rogers × | | | | | | | × © *2001 Wisconsin Dental Association*
(800) 243-4675

PATIENT'S NAME_____

Last   First   Initial

AGREEMENT TO PAY FOR DENTAL SERVICES

Agreement to Pay. For services rendered or to be rendered to me, or to others at my request, I promise to pay to Dentist $_____, plus interest and other charges as stated below ("Obligations"). I will make the payments described in the payment schedule to Dentist at the address shown on the opposite side of this form.

Federally Required Disclosures. The calculations shown below are computed on the assumption that each payment will be made in full on the date due:

ITEMIZATION OF AMOUNT FINANCED

Dental Fees   Down Payment   Amount Financed

$ _____ – $ _____ = $ _____

ANNUAL PERCENTAGE RATE	FINANCE CHARGE	Amount Financed	Total of Payments	Total Sale Price
The cost of your credit as a yearly rate.	The dollar amount the credit will cost you.	The amount of credit provided to you or on your behalf.	The amount you will have paid after you have made all payments as scheduled.	The total cost of your purchase on credit, including your downpayment of $_____
_____%	$ _____	$ _____	$ _____	$ _____

Your payment schedule will be: _____ equal consecutive installments of $ _____ each, and one final installment of _____ on the _____ day of each successive month beginning_____ , 19_____.

Late Charge. If a payment is not paid on or before the 10th day after the due date, I may be charged _____ or 5.00% of the unpaid amount, whichever is less.

If I pay off early, I will not have to pay a penalty, and I may be entitled to a refund of unearned finance charge.

See your contract documents for any additional information about nonpayments, default, any required repayment before the scheduled date, and prepayment refunds and penalties.

Other Charges. I agree to pay a charge of _____ for each check presented for payment and returned unpaid. I also agree to pay all costs of collection, to the extent not prohibited under law.

Application of Payments. Unless otherwise required by applicable law, payment will be applied as directed by Dentist.

Default and Remedies. I will be in default of my Obligations under this Agreement if I have an amount outstanding which exceeds one full payment which has remained unpaid for more than 10 days after the scheduled or deferred due dates; or the first or last payment is not paid within 40 days of its due date.

In the event of default, the Dentist shall:
   A. Have all the rights and remedies provided by law and this Agreement. All remedies shall be cumulative and __ the exercise of one shall not prevent the exercise of other remedies.
   B. Upon default the Dentist may, at his option, accelerate the amount due, without notice. In that event, the Obligations shall become payable after notice is provided and the right to cure has expired.

Miscellaneous.
   A. To the extent any provision of this Agreement is void or prohibited under applicable law, that provision shall be null and void and severed from the other terms of this Agreement. The remaining provisions shall be enforced to the fullest extent possible.
   B. The Dentist's waiver of one default does not waive any other default, whether the same or different, in the future.
   C. This Agreement is intended as the entire Agreement and replaces all prior and contemporaneous, written or oral, Agreements on the subject matter covered herein. The Agreement may only be modified by a written document signed by all parties to this Agreement.
   D. The terms "I", "me" and "my" includes each person who signs this Agreement, except the Dentist. If more than one person has signed this Agreement, each will be responsible for repaying the Obligations in full.

   I have received a copy of this Agreement.

NOTICE TO CUSTOMER	(a)	DO NOT SIGN THIS BEFORE YOU READ THE WRITING ON THE REVERSE SIDE, EVEN IF OTHERWISE ADVISED.
	(b)	DO NOT SIGN THIS IF IT CONTAINS ANY BLANK SPACES.
	(c)	YOU ARE ENTITLED TO AN EXACT COPY OF ANY AGREEMENT YOU SIGN.
	(d)	YOU HAVE THE RIGHT AT ANY TIME TO PAY IN ADVANCE THE UNPAID BALANCE DUE UNDER THIS AGREEMENT AND YOU MAY BE ENTITLED TO A PARTIAL REFUND OF FINANCE CHARGE.

Dated _____   X _____
                                                     Patient or patient's parent or legal guardian

_____   • _____
              Dentist   Print name

By _____   X _____ /
         Authorized Signature
Address: _____   • _____
                                                                  Print name
_____   Address: _____

_____

                                              County: _____

Form No. T280FA   # FINANCIAL ARRANGEMENTS - U.S.

Angelica Green

© 2003 Wisconsin Dental Association
(800) 243-4675

PATIENT NUMBER

welcome

Date _____

Patient's Name _____ Date of Birth _____ ❑ Male ❑ Female

Last   First   Initial

If Child: Parent's Name _____

How do you wish to be addressed _____
Single ❑   Married ❑   Separated ❑   Divorced ❑   Widowed ❑   Minor ❑

Residence - Street _____

City _____ State _____ Zip _____

Business Address _____

Telephone: Res. _____ Bus. _____

Fax _____ Cell Phone # _____

eMail _____

Patient/Parent Employed By _____

Present Position _____

How Long Held _____

Spouse/Parent Name _____

Spouse Employed By _____

Present Position _____

How Long Held _____

Who is Responsible for this account _____

Drivers License No. _____

Method of Payment: Insurance ❑   Cash ❑   Credit Card ❑

Purpose of Call _____

Other Family Members in this Practice _____

_____

Whom may we thank for this referral _____

Patient/parent Social Security No. _____

Spouse/Parent Social Security No. _____

Someone to notify in case of emergency not living with you _____

_____

DENTAL INSURANCE 1ST COVERAGE

Employee Name _____ Date of Birth _____
Employer Name _____ Yrs. _____
Name of Insurance Co. _____
Address _____
_____
Telephone _____
Program or policy # _____
Social Security No. _____
Union Local or Group _____

DENTAL INSURANCE 2ND COVERAGE

Employee Name _____ Date of Birth _____
Employer Name _____ Yrs. _____
Name of Insurance Co. _____
Address _____
_____
Telephone _____
Program or policy # _____
Social Security No. _____
Union Local or Group _____

CONSENT:

I consent to the diagnostic procedures and treatment by the dentist necessary for proper dental care.

I consent to the dentist's use and disclosure of my records (or my child's records) to carry out treatment, to obtain payment, and for those activities and health care operations that are related to treatment or payment.

I consent to the disclosure of my records (or my child's records) to the following persons who are involved in my care (or my child's care) or payment for that care.

_____

_____

My consent to disclosure of records shall be effective until I revoke it in writing.

I authorize payment directly to the dentist or dental group of insurance benefits otherwise payable to me. I understand that my dental care insurance carrier or payor of my dental benefits may pay less than the actual bill for services, and that I am financially responsible for payment in full of all accounts. By signing this statement, I revoke all previous agreements to the contrary and agree to be responsible for payment of services not paid, by my dental care payor.

I attest to the accuracy of the information on this page.

PATIENT'S OR GUARDIAN'S SIGNATURE

DATE _____

Form No. T110R

REGISTRATION

Angelica Green

welcome

PATIENT NUMBER

Patient's Name _____

Last	First	Initial	Date of Birth

COMMENTS

1. Purpose of initial visit _____
   _____
2. Are you aware of a problem? _____
   _____
3. How long since your last dental visit? _____
4. What was done at that time? _____
   _____
5. Previous dentist's name _____
   Address: _____ Tel. _____
6. When was the last time your teeth were cleaned? _____

CIRCLE THE APPROPRIATE ANSWER. IF YOU DON'T KNOW THE CORRECT ANSWER, PLEASE WRITE "DON'T KNOW" ON THE LINE AFTER THE QUESTION.

7. Have you made regular visits? ....YES NO
   How often: _____
8. Were dental x-rays taken? ....YES NO
9. Have you lost any teeth or have any teeth been removed? ......YES NO
   Why? _____
10. Have they been replaced? ....YES NO
11. How have they been replaced?
    a. Fixed bridge _____ Age _____
    b. Removable bridge _____ Age _____
    c. Denture _____ Age _____
    d. Implant _____ Age _____
12. Are you unhappy with the replacement? ....YES NO
    If yes, explain _____
13. Would you like to know about permanent replacements? ......YES NO
14. Have you ever had any problems or complications with previous dental treatment? ....YES NO
    If yes, explain: _____
15. Do you clench or grind your teeth? ....YES NO
16. Does your jaw click or pop? ....YES NO
17. Have you experienced any pain or soreness in the muscles of your face or around your ear? ....YES NO
18. Do you have frequent headaches, neckaches or shoulder aches? ....YES NO
19. Does food get caught in your teeth? ....YES NO
20. Are any of your teeth sensitive to: ☐ Hot? ☐ Cold? ☐ Sweets? ☐ Pressure?
21. Do your gums bleed or hurt? ....YES NO
    When? _____
22. How often do you brush your teeth? _____ When? _____
23. Do you use dental floss? ....YES NO
    How often? _____
24. Are any of your teeth loose, tipped, shifted or chipped? ...YES NO
25. Are you unhappy with the appearance of your teeth? ....YES NO
26. How do you feel about your teeth in general? _____
27. Do you feel your breath is offensive at times? ....YES NO
28. Have you ever had gum treatment or surgery? ....YES NO
    What? _____
    Where? _____
    When? _____
29. Have you had any orthodontic work? _____
30. Have you had any unpleasant dental experiences or is there anything about dentistry that you strongly dislike? _____
31. Do you have any questions or concerns? ....YES NO

I CERTIFY THAT THE ABOVE INFORMATION IS COMPLETE AND ACCURATE

PATIENT'S / GUARDIAN'S SIGNATURE _____ DATE _____

DENTIST'S SIGNATURE _____ DATE _____

ANEST.

MED. ALERT

DENTAL HISTORY

Form No. T150DH

Angelica Green

welcome

PATIENT NUMBER

© 2004 Wisconsin Dental Association
(800) 243-4675

Patient's Name _____

Last   First   Initial   Date of Birth

CIRCLE THE APPROPRIATE ANSWER, IF YOU DON'T KNOW THE CORRECT ANSWER PLEASE WRITE "DON'T KNOW" ON THE LINE AFTER THE QUESTION

COMMENTS

1. Physician's Name_____
   Address_____
   _____ Tel:(   )_____
2. Are you under a physician's care? . . . . YES NO
   Since when_____Why _____
3. When was your last complete physical exam?_____
4. Are you taking any medication or substances? . . . . YES NO
   (If yes, please list medications in comments section or on the back of this form.)
5. Do you routinely take health related substances? (Vitamins, herbal supplements, natural products) . . YES NO
6. Are you allergic to any medications or substances? (please list) . . . . YES NO
7. Do you have any other allergies or hives? . . . . YES NO
8. Do you have any problems with penicillin, antibiotics, anesthetics
   or other medications? . . . . YES NO
9. Are you sensitive to any metals or latex? . . . . YES NO
10. Are you pregnant or suspect you may be? . . . . YES NO
11. Do you use any birth control medications? . . . . YES NO
12. Have you ever been treated for or been told you might have heart disease? . . . . . YES NO
13. Do you have a pacemaker, an artificial heart valve implant, or
    been diagnosed with mitral valve prolapse? . . . . YES NO
14. Have you ever had rheumatic fever? . . . . YES NO
15. Are you aware of any heart murmurs? . . . . YES NO
16. Do you have high or low blood pressure? (please circle) . . . . YES NO
17. Have you ever had a serious illness or major surgery? . . . . YES NO
    If so, explain_____
18. Have you ever had radiation treatment, chemo treatment for tumor
    growth or other condition? . . . . YES NO
19. Do you have inflammatory diseases, such as arthritis or rheumatism? . . . . . YES NO
20. Do you have any artificial joints/prosthesis? . . . . YES NO
21. Do you have any blood disorders, such as anemia, leukemia, etc.? . . . . . YES NO
22. Have you ever bled excessively after being cut or injured? . . . . YES NO
23. Do you have any stomach problems? . . . . YES NO
24. Do you have any kidney problems? . . . . YES NO
25. Do you have any liver problems? . . . . YES NO
26. Are you diabetic? . . . . YES NO
27. Do you have fainting or dizzy spells? . . . . YES NO
28. Do you have asthma? . . . . YES NO
29. Do you have epilepsy or seizures? . . . . YES NO
30. Do you or have you had venereal disease? . . . . YES NO
31. Have you tested HIV positive? . . . . YES NO
32. Do you have AIDS? . . . . YES NO
33. Have you had or do you test positive for hepatitis? . . . . YES NO
34. Do you or have you had T.B.? . . . . YES NO
35. Do you smoke, chew, use snuff or any other forms of tobacco? . . . . . . YES NO
36. Do you regularly consume more than one or two alcoholic beverages a day? . . YES NO
37. Do you habitually use controlled substances? . . . . YES NO
38. Have you had psychiatric treatment? . . . . YES NO
39. Have you taken any prescription drugs fenfluramine, fenfluramine combined with
    phentermine (fen-phen), dexfenfluramine (redux), or other weight loss products? . . YES NO
40. Do you have any disease condition, or problem not listed? If so, explain_____
    _____
41. Is there anything else we should know about your health that we have not covered in this form?
    _____
42. Would you like to speak to the Doctor privately about any problem? . . . . YES NO

I CERTIFY THAT THE ABOVE INFORMATION IS COMPLETE AND ACCURATE

PATIENT'S / GUARDIAN'S SIGNATURE _____ DATE_____

DENTIST'S SIGNATURE _____ DATE_____

ANEST.

MED. ALERT

Form No. T140MH

MEDICAL HISTORY

131

Appendix

Angelica Green

PATIENT NUMBER

PATIENT'S NAME _____

Last   First   Initial

RHEUMATIC FEVER	ALLERGIES	AIDS	HEPATITIS	HEART COND.	MEDICATION	ANESTHETIC	BLOOD PRESSURE	PULSE

MISSING TEETH & EXISTING RESTORATIONS

1 2 3 4 5 6 7 8 9 10 11 12 13 14 15 16

B

L

DATE _____

RIGHT   A B C D E   F G H I J   LEFT
               T S R Q P   O N M L K

L

B

32 31 30 29 28 27 26 25   24 23 22 21 20 19 18 17

PATIENT'S CHIEF COMPLAINT:

EXISTING X-RAYS   DATE

BW _____
PAN _____
FMX _____
PA _____

PROSTHESIS EVALUATION
TYPE OR AREA   DATE INSERTED

SOFT TISSUE EXAMINATION	OK

COMMENTS:

OCCLUSION   EVALUATION

TMJ EVALUATION

Right: Ⴖ Crepitus   Ⴖ Snapping/Popping
Left: Ⴖ Crepitus   Ⴖ Snapping/Popping

Tenderness to Palpation:
TMJ: Ⴖ Right   Ⴖ Left
Muscles: _____
Deviation on Closing: ____Rmm_____Lmm
Maximum Opening: _____ mm

COMMENTS:

CONDITIONS / TREATMENT INDICATED

1 2 3 4 5 6 7 8 9 10 11 12 13 14 15 16

B

L

DATE _____

RIGHT   A B C D E   F G H I J   LEFT
               T S R Q P   O N M L K

L

B

32 31 30 29 28 27 26 25   24 23 22 21 20 19 18 17

Treatment Schedule Ⴖ

SIGNATURE OF DENTIST

CLINICAL EXAMINATION

Form No. T170CE

Angelica Green

© 2001 Wisconsin Dental Association
(800) 243-4675

PATIENT'S NAME _____

Last   First   Initial   Date of Birth

DATE _____ THERAPIST _____

PROBING – Place probe as close to the contact point as possible, directed along the long axis of the tooth. Take the mesial, mid and distal measurements from the buccal aspect. Repeat for lingual aspect. Record only those measurements over 3mm.
BLEEDING – After probing each quadrant, note whether or not bleeding has occurred. Indicate the bleeding area by circling the pocket in red.
MOBILITY – Move each tooth between two instrument handles in a bucco-lingual direction and attempt to depress each tooth in its socket. Grade each tooth accordingly: 0 - Movement of less than 0.5mm; 1 - 0.5mm to 1.0mm; 2 - 1.0mm to 2.0mm; 3 - Movement of more that 2.0mm or depressible.
FURCATION – Probe from the buccal and lingual. Record accordingly: 0 - Normal; 1 - Slight; 2 - Moderate; 3 - Through and through.
RECESSION – Measure the exposed surface from the cemental enamel junction (CEJ) to the gingival crest. Enter the distance in millimeters (mm).

Periodontal charting grid for teeth 1–16 (upper) and 32–17 (lower), with rows for Pocket Depth (B/L), Mobility, Furcation, and Recession.

R   **L**

	OPTION 1 / OPTION 2	
Enter highest POCKET DEPTH score in appropriate box	☐ Any pocket depth reading from 3 to 5mm, read below	☐ Any pocket depth reading over 5mm, read below
Enter highest MOBILITY SCORE in appropriate box	☐ Any mobility of 1, read below	☐ Any mobility of 2 or 3, read below

BLEEDING — ☐ When any bleeding upon probing is noted, read below

INSTRUMENTS FOR TREATMENT SELECTION — ☐ Explanation of periodontal disease.

Locate square containing score farthest to the right and follow treatment, listed below.

Gingivitis
A. Hygienist Treatment
1. Oral Hygiene Instruction
2. Prophylaxis

Moderate Periodontitis
OPTION 1
A. Dentist or Hygienist Treatment
1. Oral Hygiene Instruction
2. Periodontal Root Planing
3. Occlusal Analysis
4. Maintenance Recall
OPTION 2
B. Referral to Periodontist

Advanced Periodontitis
OPTION 1
A. Referral to Periodontist
OPTION 2
B. Dentist Treatment
1. Oral Hygiene Instruction
2. Periodontal Root Planing
3. Occlusal Analysis
4. Periodontal Surgery
5. Splinting
6. Maintenance Recall

Form No. T181PS
PERIODONTAL SCREENING EXAMINATION

Angelica Green

PATIENT NUMBER

PATIENT'S NAME _____

| Last | First | Initial | Date |

DATE	TREATMENT PLAN	FEE	ALTERNATE TREATMENT	FEE	PROB # ASGN

RELEASE:

I accept the above treatment plan. I understand that because of unexpected circumstances, the treatment, the fees for treatment and/or the materials required as explained to me at this time, may require some changes after actual care has begun.

PATIENT'S/GUARDIAN'S SIGNATURE _____ DATE _____

| ANEST. | | MED. ALERT |

TREATMENT PLAN

Form No. T201TP

Angelica Green   × [| | | | |] ×   © 2001 Wisconsin Dental Association
(800) 243-4675

PATIENT'S NAME_____
                    Last   First   Initial

AGREEMENT TO PAY FOR DENTAL SERVICES

Agreement to Pay. For services rendered or to be rendered to me, or to others at my request, I promise to pay to Dentist $_____, plus interest and other charges as stated below ("Obligations"). I will make the payments described in the payment schedule to Dentist at the address shown on the opposite side of this form.

Federally Required Disclosures. The calculations shown below are computed on the assumption that each payment will be made in full on the date due:

ITEMIZATION OF AMOUNT FINANCED

Dental Fees   Down Payment   Amount Financed

$ _____ – $ _____ = $ _____

ANNUAL PERCENTAGE RATE	FINANCE CHARGE	Amount Financed	Total of Payments	Total Sale Price
The cost of your credit as a yearly rate.	The dollar amount the credit will cost you.	The amount of credit provided to you or on your behalf.	The amount you will have paid after you have made all payments as scheduled.	The total cost of your purchase on credit, including your downpayment of $_____
_____%	$_____	$_____	$_____	$_____

Your payment schedule will be: _____ equal consecutive installments of $ _____ each, and one final installment of _____ on the _____ day of each successive month beginning_____ , 19_____.

Late Charge. If a payment is not paid on or before the 10th day after the due date, I may be charged $ ____ or 5.00% of the unpaid amount, whichever is less.

If I pay off early, I will not have to pay a penalty, and I may be entitled to a refund of unearned finance charge.

See your contract documents for any additional information about nonpayment, default, any required repayment before the scheduled date, and prepayment refunds and penalties.

Other Charges. I agree to pay a charge of _____ for each check presented for payment and returned unpaid. I also agree to pay all costs of collection, to the extent not prohibited under law.

Application of Payments. Unless otherwise required by applicable law, payment will be applied as directed by Dentist.

Default and Remedies. I will be in default of my Obligations under this Agreement if I have an amount outstanding which exceeds one full payment which has remained unpaid for more than 10 days after the scheduled or deferred due dates; or the first or last payment is not paid within 40 days of its due date.

In the event of default, the Dentist shall:

A. Have all the rights and remedies provided by law and this Agreement. All remedies shall be cumulative and __ the exercise of one shall not prevent the exercise of any other remedies.

B. Upon default the Dentist may, at his discretion, accelerate the amount due, without notice. In that event, the Obligations shall become payable after notice is provided and the right to cure has expired.

Miscellaneous.

A. To the extent any provision of this Agreement is void or prohibited under applicable law, that provision shall be null and void and severed from the other terms of this Agreement. The remaining provisions shall be enforced to the fullest extent possible.

B. The Dentist's waiver of one default does not waive any other default, whether the same or different, in the future.

C. This Agreement is intended as the entire Agreement and replaces all prior and contemporaneous, written or oral, Agreements on the subject matter covered herein. The Agreement may only be modified by a written by all parties to this Agreement.

D. The terms "I", "me" and "my" includes each person who signs this Agreement, except the Dentist. If more than one person has signed this Agreement, each will be responsible for repaying the Obligations in full.

I have received a copy of this Agreement.

NOTICE TO CUSTOMER	(a) DO NOT SIGN THIS BEFORE YOU READ THE WRITING ON THE REVERSE SIDE, EVEN IF OTHERWISE ADVISED.
	(b) DO NOT SIGN THIS IF IT CONTAINS ANY BLANK SPACES.
	(c) YOU ARE ENTITLED TO AN EXACT COPY OF ANY AGREEMENT YOU SIGN.
	(d) YOU HAVE THE RIGHT AT ANY TIME TO PAY IN ADVANCE THE UNPAID BALANCE DUE UNDER THIS AGREEMENT AND YOU MAY BE ENTITLED TO A PARTIAL REFUND OF FINANCE CHARGE.

Dated _____   X _____
                                              Patient or patient's parent or legal guardian
                                            • _____
_____   _____
             Dentist   Print name

By _____   X _____ /
           Authorized Signature
Address: _____   • _____
                                                Print name
_____   Address: _____

                                        _____

                                        County: _____

FINANCIAL ARRANGEMENTS - U.S.

Form No. T280FA

135

Holly Barry

| | | | | | |

PATIENT NUMBER

welcome

Date _____

Patient's Name _____   Date of Birth _____ ☐ Male ☐ Female
Last   First   Initial

If Child: Parent's Name _____

How do you wish to be addressed _____
Single ☐   Married ☐   Separated ☐   Divorced ☐   Widowed ☐   Minor ☐

Residence - Street _____

City _____ State _____ Zip _____

Business Address _____

Telephone: Res. _____ Bus. _____

Fax _____ Cell Phone # _____

eMail _____

Patient/Parent Employed By _____

Present Position _____

How Long Held _____

Spouse/Parent Name _____

Spouse Employed By _____

Present Position _____

How Long Held _____

Who is Responsible for this account _____

Drivers License No. _____

Method of Payment: Insurance ☐   Cash ☐   Credit Card ☐

Purpose of Call _____

Other Family Members in this Practice _____

_____

Whom may we thank for this referral _____

Patient/parent Social Security No. _____

Spouse/Parent Social Security No. _____

Someone to notify in case of emergency not living with you _____

_____

DENTAL INSURANCE 1ST COVERAGE

Employee Name _____ Date of Birth _____
Employer Name _____ Yrs. _____
Name of Insurance Co. _____
Address _____
_____
Telephone _____
Program or policy # _____
Social Security No. _____
Union Local or Group _____

DENTAL INSURANCE 2ND COVERAGE

Employee Name _____ Date of Birth _____
Employer Name _____ Yrs. _____
Name of Insurance Co. _____
Address _____
_____
Telephone _____
Program or policy # _____
Social Security No. _____
Union Local or Group _____

CONSENT:
I consent to the diagnostic procedures and treatment by the dentist necessary for proper dental care.

I consent to the dentist's use and disclosure of my records (or my child's records) to carry out treatment, to obtain payment, and for those activities and health care operations that are related to treatment or payment.

I consent to the disclosure of my records (or my child's records) to the following persons who are involved in my care (or my child's care) or payment for that care.

_____

My consent to disclosure of records shall be effective until I revoke it in writing.

I authorize payment directly to the dentist or dental group of insurance benefits otherwise payable to me. I understand that my dental care insurance carrier or payor of my dental benefits may pay less than the actual bill for services, and that I am financially responsible for payment in full of all accounts. By signing this statement, I revoke all previous agreements to the contrary and agree to be responsible for payment of services not paid, by my dental care payor.

I attest to the accuracy of the information on this page.

PATIENT'S OR GUARDIAN'S SIGNATURE

DATE _____

Form No. T110R

REGISTRATION

Holly Barry

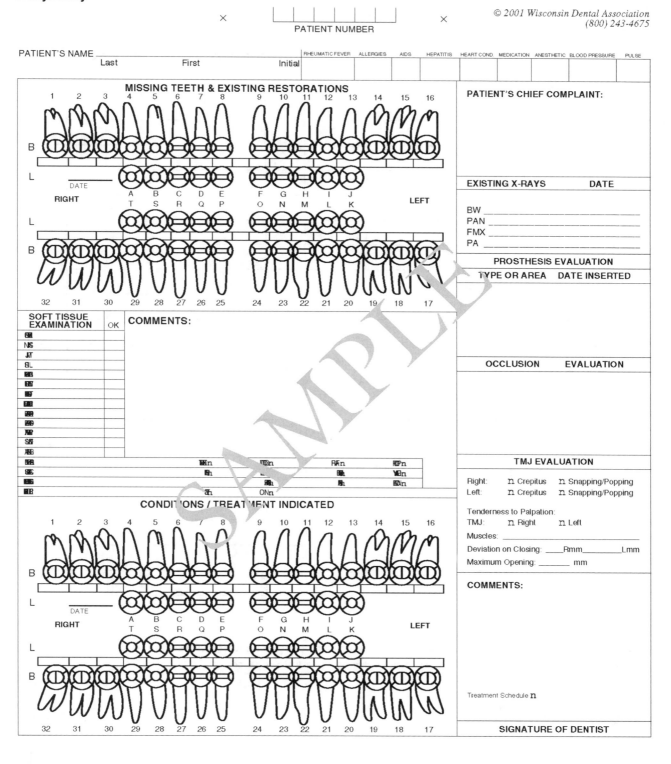

× PATIENT NUMBER ×

PATIENT'S NAME _____
Last   First   Initial

RHEUMATIC FEVER	ALLERGIES	AIDS	HEPATITIS	HEART COND.	MEDICATION	ANESTHETIC	BLOOD PRESSURE	PULSE

MISSING TEETH & EXISTING RESTORATIONS

1 2 3 4 5 6 7 8 9 10 11 12 13 14 15 16

B

L

DATE _____
RIGHT   A B C D E   F G H I J   LEFT
             T S R Q P   O N M L K

L

B

32 31 30 29 28 27 26 25 24 23 22 21 20 19 18 17

PATIENT'S CHIEF COMPLAINT:

EXISTING X-RAYS   DATE

BW _____
PAN _____
FMX _____
PA _____

PROSTHESIS EVALUATION
TYPE OR AREA   DATE INSERTED

SOFT TISSUE EXAMINATION	OK

COMMENTS:

OCCLUSION   EVALUATION

TMJ EVALUATION

Right: n Crepitus   n Snapping/Popping
Left: n Crepitus   n Snapping/Popping

Tenderness to Palpation:
TMJ: n Right   n Left
Muscles: _____
Deviation on Closing: ____Rmm_____Lmm
Maximum Opening: _____ mm

CONDITIONS / TREATMENT INDICATED

1 2 3 4 5 6 7 8 9 10 11 12 13 14 15 16

B

L

DATE _____
RIGHT   A B C D E   F G H I J   LEFT
             T S R Q P   O N M L K

L

B

32 31 30 29 28 27 26 25 24 23 22 21 20 19 18 17

COMMENTS:

Treatment Schedule n

SIGNATURE OF DENTIST

CLINICAL EXAMINATION

Form No. T170CE

Holly Barry

PATIENT NUMBER

PATIENT'S NAME _____

| | Last | First | Initial | Date | |

DATE	TREATMENT PLAN	FEE	ALTERNATE TREATMENT	FEE	PROB # ASGN

RELEASE:

I accept the above treatment plan. I understand that because of unexpected circumstances, the treatment, the fees for treatment and/or the materials required as explained to me at this time, may require some changes after actual care has begun.

PATIENT'S/GUARDIAN'S SIGNATURE _____ DATE _____

ANEST.		MED. ALERT

Form No. T201TP

TREATMENT PLAN

Holly Barry × | | | | | | × © 2001 Wisconsin Dental Association
(800) 243-4675

PATIENT'S NAME_____

| Last | First | Initial |

AGREEMENT TO PAY FOR DENTAL SERVICES

Agreement to Pay. For services rendered or to be rendered to me, or to others at my request, I promise to pay to Dentist $_____, plus interest and other charges as stated below ("Obligations"). I will make the payments described in the payment schedule to Dentist at the address shown on the opposite side of this form.

Federally Required Disclosures. The calculations shown below are computed on the assumption that each payment will be made in full on the date due:

ITEMIZATION OF AMOUNT FINANCED

| Dental Fees | Down Payment | Amount Financed |

$_____ – $_____ = $_____

| ANNUAL PERCENTAGE RATE

The cost of your credit as a yearly rate.

_____% | FINANCE CHARGE

The dollar amount the credit will cost you.

$_____ | Amount Financed

The amount of credit provided to you or on your behalf.

$_____ | Total of Payments

The amount you will have paid after you have made all payments as scheduled.

$_____ | Total Sale Price

The total cost of your purchase on credit, including your downpayment of
$_____
$_____ |

Your payment schedule will be: _____ equal consecutive installments of $ _____ each. and one final installment of _____ on the _____ day of each successive month beginning_____, 19_____.

Late Charge. If a payment is not paid on or before the 10th day after the due date, I may be charged $_____ or 5.00% of the _____ paid amount, whichever is less.

If I pay off early, I will not have to pay a penalty, and I may be entitled to a refund of unearned finance charge.

See your contract documents for any additional information about nonpayments, default, any required repayment _____ before the scheduled date, and prepayment refunds and penalties.

Other Charges. I agree to pay a charge of _____ for each check pr_____nted for paym_nt and returned unpaid. I also agree to pay all costs of collection, to the extent not pr_____ under la_.

Application of Payments. Unless otherwise required _ applicable law, paymen_ _l be applied as directed by Dentist.

Default and Remedies. I will be in default of _y Obligations _der this Agreement if I have an amount outstanding which exceeds one full payment which has r_ined unpaid fo_ _re than 10 days after the scheduled or deferred due dates; or the first or last payment is not pai_ _n 40 days of _ _ date.

In the event of default, the Dentist shall:
A. Have all the rights and reme_ies provided _ law a_ _his Agreement. All remedies shall be cumulative and __ the exercise of one shall n_ _nt the exe_cise of _ other remedies.

B. Upon default the Dentist may, _t his _ _ion, accelerate the amount due, without notice. In that event, the Obligations shall become pay_le after n_ _e is provided and the right to cure has expired.

Miscellaneous.
A. To the extent a_y _ _ion of this Ag_ _ment is void or prohibited under applicable law, that provision shall be null and voi_ and s_ _ from t_e other terms of this Agreement. The remaining provisions shall be enforced to the fu_est _xtent _ _e.
B. The _entist's waiv_ of one de_ult does not waive any other default, whether the same or different, in the future.
C. This Agreement is i_ended as the entire Agreement and replaces all prior and contemporaneous, written or _ral, Agreements on _ _subject matter covered herein. The Agreement may only be modified by a written _ _by a_ parties to this Agreement.
D. The _erms "I", _ _" and "my" includes each person who signs this Agreement, except the Dentist. If more than one perso_ has signed this Agreement, each will be responsible for repaying the Obligations in full.

I have re_ _d a copy of this Agreement.

NOTICE TO CUSTOMER	(a)	DO NOT SIGN THIS BEFORE YOU READ THE WRITING ON THE REVERSE SIDE, EVEN IF OTHERWISE ADVISED.
	(b)	DO NOT SIGN THIS IF IT CONTAINS ANY BLANK SPACES.
	(c)	YOU ARE ENTITLED TO AN EXACT COPY OF ANY AGREEMENT YOU SIGN.
	(d)	YOU HAVE THE RIGHT AT ANY TIME TO PAY IN ADVANCE THE UNPAID BALANCE DUE UNDER THIS AGREEMENT AND YOU MAY BE ENTITLED TO A PARTIAL REFUND OF FINANCE CHARGE.

Dated _____   X_____
_____   Patient or patient's parent or legal guardian
      Dentist   •
By _____   _____
      Authorized Signature   Print name
Address: _____   X_____ /
_____   •
                           _____
                              Print name
                           Address: _____
                           _____
                           County: _____

Form No. T280FA   **FINANCIAL ARRANGEMENTS - U.S.**

Lynn Bacca

welcome

PATIENT NUMBER

Date _____

Patient's Name _____   Date of Birth _____ ❑ Male ❑ Female
          Last   First   Initial

If Child: Parent's Name _____

How do you wish to be addressed _____
Single ❑   Married ❑   Separated ❑   Divorced ❑   Widowed ❑   Minor ❑

Residence - Street _____

City _____ State _____ Zip _____

Business Address _____

Telephone: Res. _____ Bus. _____

Fax _____ Cell Phone # _____

eMail _____

Patient/Parent Employed By _____

Present Position _____

How Long Held _____

Spouse/Parent Name _____

Spouse Employed By _____

Present Position _____

How Long Held _____

Who is Responsible for this account _____

Drivers License No. _____

Method of Payment: Insurance ❑   Cash ❑   Credit Card ❑

Purpose of Call _____

Other Family Members in this Practice _____

_____

Whom may we thank for this referral _____

Patient/parent Social Security No. _____

Spouse/Parent Social Security No. _____

Someone to notify in case of emergency not living with you _____

_____

DENTAL INSURANCE 1ST COVERAGE

Employee Name _____ Date of Birth _____
Employer Name _____ Yrs. _____
Name of Insurance Co. _____
Address _____
_____
Telephone _____
Program or policy # _____
Social Security No. _____
Union Local or Group _____

DENTAL INSURANCE 2ND COVERAGE

Employee Name _____ Date of Birth _____
Employer Name _____ Yrs. _____
Name of Insurance Co. _____
Address _____
_____
Telephone _____
Program or policy # _____
Social Security No. _____
Union Local or Group _____

CONSENT:

I consent to the diagnostic procedures and treatment by the dentist necessary for proper dental care.

I consent to the dentist's use and disclosure of my records (or my child's records) to carry out treatment, to obtain payment, and for those activities and health care operations that are related to treatment or payment.

I consent to the disclosure of my records (or my child's records) to the following persons who are involved in my care (or my child's care) or payment for that care.

_____

My consent to disclosure of records shall be effective until I revoke it in writing.

I authorize payment directly to the dentist or dental group of insurance benefits otherwise payable to me. I understand that my dental care insurance carrier or payor of my dental benefits may pay less than the actual bill for services, and that I am financially responsible for payment in full of all accounts. By signing this statement, I revoke all previous agreements to the contrary and agree to be responsible for payment of services not paid, by my dental care payor.

I attest to the accuracy of the information on this page.

PATIENT'S OR GUARDIAN'S SIGNATURE

_____

DATE _____

Form No. T110R

REGISTRATION

Lynn Bacca

× | | | | | | | | ×
PATIENT NUMBER

PATIENT'S NAME _____
Last   First   Initial

RHEUMATIC FEVER	ALLERGIES	AIDS	HEPATITIS	HEART COND.	MEDICATION	ANESTHETIC	BLOOD PRESSURE	PULSE

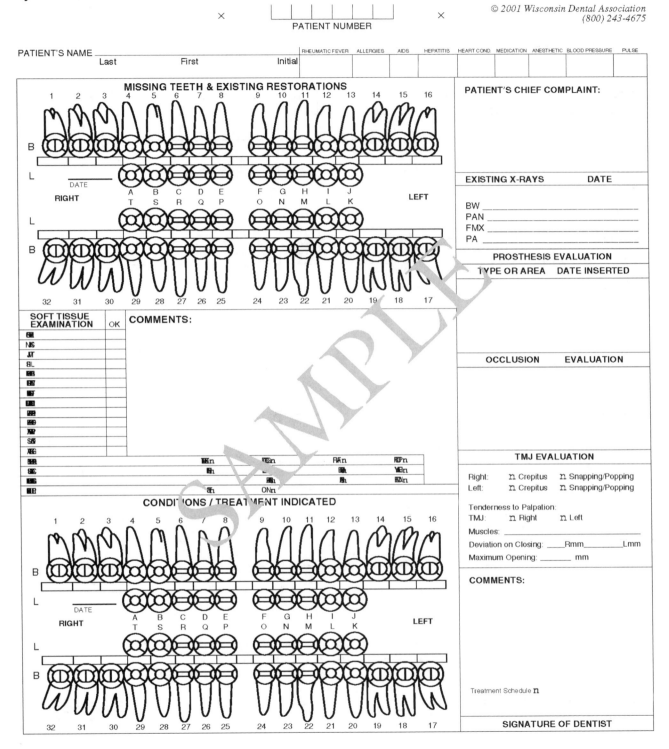

MISSING TEETH & EXISTING RESTORATIONS

PATIENT'S CHIEF COMPLAINT:

EXISTING X-RAYS   DATE

BW _____
PAN _____
FMX _____
PA _____

PROSTHESIS EVALUATION
TYPE OR AREA   DATE INSERTED

OCCLUSION   EVALUATION

SOFT TISSUE EXAMINATION   OK

COMMENTS:

TMJ EVALUATION

Right: n Crepitus   n Snapping/Popping
Left: n Crepitus   n Snapping/Popping

Tenderness to Palpation:
TMJ: n Right   n Left
Muscles: _____
Deviation on Closing: ____Rmm_____Lmm
Maximum Opening: _____ mm

COMMENTS:

CONDITIONS / TREATMENT INDICATED

Treatment Schedule n

SIGNATURE OF DENTIST

Form No. T170CE

CLINICAL EXAMINATION

Lynn Bacca

PATIENT NUMBER

PATIENT'S NAME _____

| | Last | | First | | Initial | | Date | |

DATE	TREATMENT PLAN	FEE	ALTERNATE TREATMENT	FEE	PROB # ASGN

RELEASE:

I accept the above treatment plan. I understand that because of unexpected circumstances, the treatment, the fees for treatment and/or the materials required as explained to me at this time, may require some changes after actual care has begun.

PATIENT'S/GUARDIAN'S SIGNATURE _____ DATE _____

| ANEST. |

| MED. ALERT |

Form No. T201TP

TREATMENT PLAN

Lynn Bacca ✕ | | | | | | | ✕ © 2001 Wisconsin Dental Association
(800) 243-4675

PATIENT'S NAME_____

| Last | First | Initial |

AGREEMENT TO PAY FOR DENTAL SERVICES

Agreement to Pay. For services rendered or to be rendered to me, or to others at my request, I promise to pay to Dentist $_____, plus interest and other charges as stated below ("Obligations"). I will make the payments described in the payment schedule to Dentist at the address shown on the opposite side of this form.

Federally Required Disclosures. The calculations shown below are computed on the assumption that each payment will be made in full on the date due:

ITEMIZATION OF AMOUNT FINANCED

| Dental Fees | Down Payment | Amount Financed |

$ _____ – $ _____ = $ _____

ANNUAL PERCENTAGE RATE	FINANCE CHARGE	Amount Financed	Total of Payments	Total Sale Price
The cost of your credit as a yearly rate.	The dollar amount the credit will cost you.	The amount of credit provided to you or on your behalf.	The amount you will have paid after you have made all payments as scheduled.	The total cost of your purchase on credit, including your downpayment of $_____
_____%	$_____	$_____	$_____	$_____

Your payment schedule will be: _____ equal consecutive installments of $ _____ each, and one final installment of _____ on the _____ day of each successive month beginning_____ , 19_____.

Late Charge. If a payment is not paid on or before the 10th day after the due date, I may be charged ___ or 5.00% of the unpaid amount, whichever is less.

If I pay off early, I will not have to pay a penalty, and I may be entitled to a refund of unearned finance charge.

See your contract documents for any additional information about nonpayments, default, any required repayment before the scheduled date, and prepayment refunds and penalties.

Other Charges. I agree to pay a charge of _____ for each check presented for payment and returned unpaid. I also agree to pay all costs of collection, to the extent not prohibited under law.

Application of Payments. Unless otherwise required by applicable law, payments will be applied as directed by Dentist.

Default and Remedies. I will be in default of my Obligations under this Agreement if I have an amount outstanding which exceeds one full payment which has remained unpaid for more than 10 days after the scheduled or deferred due dates; or the first or last payment is not paid within 40 days of its date.

In the event of default, the Dentist shall:

    A. Have all the rights and remedies provided by law and this Agreement. All remedies shall be cumulative and ___ the exercise of one shall prevent the exercise of any other remedies.

    B. Upon default the Dentist may, at his option, accelerate the amount due, without notice. In that event, the Obligations shall become payable after notice is provided and the right to cure has expired.

Miscellaneous.

    A. To the extent any provision of this Agreement is void or prohibited under applicable law, that provision shall be null and void and severed from the other terms of this Agreement. The remaining provisions shall be enforced to the fullest extent possible.

    B. The Dentist's waiver of one default does not waive any other default, whether the same or different, in the future.

    C. This Agreement is intended as the entire Agreement and replaces all prior and contemporaneous, written or oral, Agreements on the subject matter covered herein. The Agreement may only be modified by a written document signed by all parties to this Agreement.

    D. The terms "I", "me" and "my" includes each person who signs this Agreement, except the Dentist. If more than one person has signed this Agreement, each will be responsible for repaying the Obligations in full.

    I have received a copy of this Agreement.

NOTICE TO CUSTOMER	(a)	DO NOT SIGN THIS BEFORE YOU READ THE WRITING ON THE REVERSE SIDE, EVEN IF OTHERWISE ADVISED.
	(b)	DO NOT SIGN THIS IF IT CONTAINS ANY BLANK SPACES.
	(c)	YOU ARE ENTITLED TO AN EXACT COPY OF ANY AGREEMENT YOU SIGN.
	(d)	YOU HAVE THE RIGHT AT ANY TIME TO PAY IN ADVANCE THE UNPAID BALANCE DUE UNDER THIS AGREEMENT AND YOU MAY BE ENTITLED TO A PARTIAL REFUND OF FINANCE CHARGE.

Dated _____   X _____

_____   Patient or patient's parent or legal guardian

           Dentist   • _____

By _____   X _____ /

         Authorized Signature   Print name

Address: _____   • _____

                                        Print name

_____   Address: _____

   County: _____

Form No. T280FA   **FINANCIAL ARRANGEMENTS - U.S.**